Lizzie
Gardner

The Beauty
of Me

IW
Press

First Published in Great Britain by IW Press Ltd

Author photo – author's own
Cover design by Iain Hill, 1981D
Interior design by Catherine Williams, Chapter One Book Design

A catalogue record of this book is available from the British Library.

ISBN-13: 978-1-916701-14-4 (Paperback)
ISBN-13: 978-1-916701-15-1 (e-book)

https://www.iliffe-wood.co.uk/
62-64 Market Street
Ashby-de-la-Zouch
England
LE65 1AN

Love for *The Beauty of Me*

This personal memoire is written as snippets of key moments, experiences and memories throughout the authors life. It is refreshingly non-judgemental and non-blaming, accepting feelings as one of the many things that change over time as part of life's rich tapestry.

As a woman in her 50s, like the author, it led me to reflect on the differences in values, attitudes and behaviours of our parents' generation, and made me think of my own upbringing. Comparing and contrasting some of my own experiences of being parented reminded me of the important role these sometimes everyday-experiences had in shaping my own inner world.

It highlights the juxtaposition of external versus internal worlds, and the negative impact of pressure within society leading to prioritising outward appearances. There is a vulnerability and honesty in the detail that, as a woman, I could totally relate to.

Dr Eleanor Rowsell, Consultant Clinical Psychologist

I have known Liz for over 20 years and thought I knew her well, and yet I have learned so much more about her from this book. It is well constructed, bite sized chunks, and draws us in as each of her stories are so relatable to everyone. I thought I would read it over a few days, as I usually read books, but this book drew me in, made me curious to learn more, and to my surprise I finished it all in just one day.

Liz's story is one of overcoming challenges and facing up to adversity. She shows us that every one of us has courage and wisdom at our core, and that we too can conquer far more than we ever imagine. With this, Liz is an inspiration to us all. Thank you Liz for sharing your story with the world.

Antony Tinker, Founder, iTS-Leadership Ltd

Many people feel pressure, both internal and external, to *look* beautiful on the outside. Sadly, this often hides the real beauty that lies within. Lizzie's collection of 'moments' from her life takes the reader on this journey of self-discovery to reveal her own inner beauty. It is also a story of courage, determination, resilience and hope, that we can all relate to. Writing down our experiences gives us an opportunity to reflect on them, and the simple structure of short stories is something that everyone can emulate to uncover their own beauty within.

Ursula Clare Franklin, author of *Mission Penguin,*
a photographic quest from the Galápagos to
Antarctica **(Bloomsbury Wildlife, 2024)**

A beautifully honest book showing how the author discovers her inner strength and resilience. I resonated with so much of the story; the challenges of adolescence, the search for a place in the world, losing yourself in the trappings of life and facing up to the loss of loved ones. Once started, it was very hard to put down. I highly recommend it to anyone ready for a nudge to remember that life is a gift and to rediscover the beauty in themselves.

Christine Mander, Writer and Alexander Technique Teacher

In *The Beauty of Me*, Lizzie Gardner uses snapshots in time, moments of understanding and recognition that, when taken together, paint a picture of a life well-lived. Bite-sized chapters evoke the playfulness of childhood and the tumult of adolescence, the highs and lows of love, and the terrifying confrontation of mortality. Gardner's collection of recollections – some vivid, some merely hinting at what lurks beneath – reads like a conversation with friends, shared moments of connection and understanding.

Dina Honour, Writer and Author of *It's a Lot*
to Unpack **and** *There's Some Place Like Home*

In *The Beauty of Me*, Liz does something that many of us avoid: taking an unflinching look in the mirror. This raw and honest examination of her life is as readable as it is relatable and, almost without realising it, her readers will find themselves thinking about the experiences and relationships that have shaped them too. A thought-provoking read which proves that even life's greatest challenges can have a positive purpose.

Sara Balme, Copywriter

The Beauty of Me had me captivated from the start as I found myself immersed in Lizzie's journey, feeling the ups, downs, joys and heartaches through her honest and heartfelt depiction of her life. Lizzie's determination and self-belief in the face of life-changing challenges is truly inspirational, navigating every hurdle with integrity, courage and an ever-present sense of humour! This book has taught me that no matter what curve balls life may throw our way, we all have a beauty within us.

Kate Mathur, Writer

The will to live, the love to herself shines through on every page.

Rob Hollows

There is something in *The Beauty of Me* that will resonate with us all.
   It feels so honest and heartfelt.
   Whether it be childhood camping trips, first loves, divorce, or watching loved ones battle with illness.
   It makes you consider your own life, your own truths and your own happiness.

Pam Lawson, Teacher

The Beauty of Me is not just a memoir. It's a celebration of life. A story of triumph over adversity. A mirror of the beauty we all have inside.

Lizzie's story made me laugh out loud, cry and reflect on my own journey.

This brave woman demonstrates how we all have the power to face what life throws at us and not just survive but **thrive**.

Jacqueline Hollows, Social Entrepreneur and Author
of *Wing of an Angel* and *Let Them Feel It*

Dedication

For Billy and Lexi
My Two Best Friends

Table of Contents

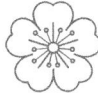

The 'Moment'

April 2024, Southern Thailand

Cancer was cruel
Cancer was a gift
Forget about me and love the 'moment'
I don't care about the past
I can't think about the future
The moment is now
This second, this minute, this hour, this day…
absorbs me
delights me
scares me
The 'moment' makes my heart sing,
My eyes dance and shine,
flash like bright flickering mirrors that record every detail
Life is a miracle and a gift
I only have now
I only have the moment

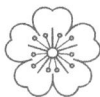

Prologue

The Operating Theatre

August 2023

"I refuse to look and act ill," I said.

I almost skipped to the sterile green operating theatre on a warm August morning, Bill by my side. He was sweating. His eyes were darting at a rapid speed, a sure sign he was as nervous as I was. We were trying to convince ourselves, and each other, that we had this under control.

What if I die?

I looked down at my new fluffy white slippers and felt the heaviness of the luxurious faux fur cream dressing gown I had brought for the occasion. It was all about looking right and being seen to be OK.

My mind drifted back to the seriousness of the operation.

Of course I wouldn't die. I would be fine.

I felt too well to be sick. I had way too much to live for. I paused at the large swing doors. I reached out for Bill, for the feel of his warm muscular arms around my tiny, bony shoulders. "I'll see you later honey," I said, forcing a smile and tossing my hair back with fake confidence.

"Love you baby," I said. I stared ahead into the pre-operative suite, not able to look into his scared eyes. It was too much. My heart was breaking.

Bill was gone, and I was alone.

My body has to get through this. It just bloody well has to.

I removed my dressing gown, climbed onto the trolley and lay back. The theatre sister squeezed my trembling hand.

Part One

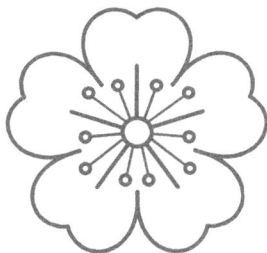

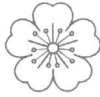

Chapter 1

First Memory

August 1973, my fifth birthday

The thrill of my party had worn off. Fast.

I hated the squabbles, the arguments about who should sit next to whom, who had the prettiest dress. There'd been spilt cream soda, copious amounts of jelly and ice cream, and hot tears of excitement and tantrums. I didn't like being in the limelight. I liked the thought of it, but not the reality. I had made my escape.

Long tanned five-year-old legs sprinted up the narrow-manicured lawn. I squeezed under the padlocked gate with no regard for the cream and brown daisy dress I wore; the smocked frock that Grandma and Mum had picked out for me. The one that would be passed on to my little sister the next year and then quilted into a bedspread the year after that.

I crawled into an immaculate, large vegetable area. I flopped down, heavy as a sack of potatoes under unruly rhubarb leaves. I shut my eyes and wished everyone would go away. I'd had enough. I had wanted the day to be all about me, but now my eyes stung with tiredness. I wanted the soft fragrant soil to swallow me up and take me to the land of sweet deep sleep. All year, I had counted down to the big day and now I wanted to drown out the noise and just get on with being five.

My official name is Elizabeth Ann. Libby to my little sister, and Liz, or Lizzie, to my friends. "Like the Queen," my mum always said. Granny told me I was named after the popular 1950s kitchen furniture range! Mum had told me I was going to be a Louise, or James, if I had been a boy. They changed their mind when I was born because I didn't look like a Louise.

I wanted to be called Andrea – a sophisticated name. I used to play at being Andrea. I imagined my Andrea-self had been adopted into this family. She was posh. She could have been royal. In my five-year-old head, Andrea had long blonde hair, was modern, had a horse, an apartment in London overlooking Regents Park and a bright yellow convertible car. She also had lots of friends and knew what to do in any situation. She was confident. Sassy.

I named my favourite Sindy doll Andrea. She went everywhere with me. I dressed her each day, a different outfit for every occasion. I combed and cleaned her hair until it shone a bright platinum blonde – a very different look to my sister's Sindy who was neglected, had matted brown hair and was missing a leg.

My sister, Jane, and I were like North and South. She climbed trees, collected spiders, ate mud, didn't care for anything pink or furry, and had a fear of water and hairbrushes.

We could be thick as thieves or arch enemies. We each thought the other was our parents' favourite. Whilst some of her antics seemed fearless, Jane had an inner fragility the whole family looked out for. Two years younger than me, she got more attention and was referred to as the baby of the family. She also got the bigger bedroom! That didn't feel fair. Mum said she needed the extra space, seeing as she was a natural collector of stuff.

All I wanted was to be loved, to get things right, and for my parents to be proud of me. My five-year-old head would ache as, curled up on a beanbag in my tiny bedroom, my mind would spin with ideas designed to make Mum and Dad proud. I tried to work out how to be the apple of their eye, their pride and joy. Even at five years of age, there seemed to be a high expectation for perfection, and I was falling short. The older I got, the higher and higher the bar got.

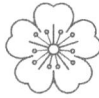

Chapter 2

Love and Innocence

"Girls, please do not lean on the sides of the tent, the rain will leak in," barked my father at my sister and I.

"Really Dad?" we would mutter with frustration.

Why were we camping in the Highlands of Scotland in the middle of August, we would question our parents until we were blue in the face.

Why couldn't we be like normal families and holiday in a hotel in Majorca, or a villa in Portugal? We didn't like being different.

"Are we poor?" we would ask Mum and Dad.

"No," was the stock answer. "We want to bring you up with an appreciation of the British Isles and its beautiful nature and wildlife."

We had never been abroad. We spent our school holidays in Scotland, the Lake District, Wales, Dorset, or, for a bit of variety, Devon or Cornwall.

The summer of 1978 was a Scottish one. A camping trip to the Inner Hebridean Isle of Mull.

The rains had been heavy that year. Our dated, dark blue family ridge tent had blown down on more than one occasion. It seemed impossible to keep the gas ring on our small burner alight for more than a couple of minutes. What a shock we had when we returned from a village ceilidh one evening to find the tent down, blown flat, our belongings scattered across the field.

Even that didn't grant us a meal out, or a night's stay in a hotel.

Normal families went out for meals in restaurants and pubs, yet we had to heat everything up straight from the can.

Our meals consisted of some kind of meat product, mince, meatballs or sausages, with Smash potato. Smash was an easy choice for camping: dried potato granules mixed with hot water to make mash. It was disgusting. Jane and I hated it.

There was a certain wholesome innocence about our holidays. Utter freedom. The challenge of being self-sufficient in the wilderness. The wildlife lessons from Dad were relentless, but we were rewarded with daily sightings of deer, otter, reptiles, birds, and dolphins.

To be cool, we appeared to be unimpressed by these rare sightings, but Jane and I couldn't conceal our excitement and were both proud owners of binoculars. We led the way in our peer group conversations when it came to UK geography and wildlife; precious insights that keep giving to this very day.

In late 1978, we had a breakthrough. Not quite a hotel, but a cottage to rent.

Wow! That had been music to our young, hopeful ears.

A colleague of Dad's had inherited a rustic stone bungalow,

overlooking the Mawddach Estuary in North Wales. Originally a gatehouse to a Victorian Manor House, it was small, yet proud. It was a white rendered building with a black framed, traditional bay window, a slate roof and Victorian wrought iron railings at the front. The magnificent views across the estuary and mountain range beyond were breathtaking.

To say it was basic is an understatement, but it was our basic and we loved it. It beat canvas any day.

Inside, it had a cozy lounge with an open fireplace, a two-seater sofa, and two dark green leather armchairs at either side of the fire. In the corner of the lounge stood an enormous Welsh dresser, carved in oak with an intricate finish, displaying a collection of Willow pattern plates. Although the dresser dominated the room, and was way too big for the space, its history fascinated Jane and I. We guessed it had once sat pride of place in the drawing room of the grand manor house, at the top of the drive.

Off the lounge was a tiny kitchen with an ancient Aga and an original stone floor. To our bare feet first thing in the morning, it was like walking on an ice rink. There were two bedrooms, a double, and a twin. The beds were ancient with hard, lumpy mattresses and dusty iron frames. We didn't care as we snuggled deep inside our cozy sleeping bags. Mum always took plenty of blankets and hot water bottles, in case we got cold. There was no hot running water in the kitchen or the bathroom, and each morning we had to boil kettles to wash.

Despite its limitations and rustic style, to us, it was beautiful. Our palace. A place we migrated back to every spring and autumn half-term for over ten years.

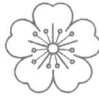

Chapter 3

Where did Dad go?

My dad had always been my hero, my immediate go-to in any situation – good, bad, exciting or scary.

When I was four or five years old, I would stand in the front porch each evening, knowing Dad would walk through the door at 6 pm sharp. He would lift me up, wrap me with love in the firm grasp of his long arms, while my legs dangled freely.

I felt safe.

I would barely give him time to get his jacket off before asking him if I could practice my reading or beg him to give me an elephant ride on his back around our living room.

I loved Dad so much. He was my favourite parent. He had been my world.

My love for Dad came with implicit trust and respect.

He was clever – a natural academic – one of those people who could turn their hand to anything. If we needed a new kitchen, he would fit it. When the central heating broke down, he would repair it. When the car needed servicing, he would do it himself. We would often joke that for someone so academic, he had also been blessed with a practical gene, unlike me and Mum, who couldn't fit or repair anything!

He was great fun and had a genuine interest in people. He was well-liked and respected at the hospital where he worked as a senior microbiologist in the research laboratories.

I had been proud to talk about him to my school friends and, with great fondness, I can recall many a playground conversation around topics like "What does your dad do?" "What car does your dad drive?"

I was as proud as punch that my dad put on a white coat each day and that we had the latest Morris Marina parked on our drive, even if the colour was diarrhoea brown as my sister used to call it!

Sometimes, if I was lucky, Dad would take me into the hospital on a Saturday morning. He would lift me up onto one of the high laboratory benches. He was patient as I conducted mini experiments. With curious young eyes, my small, gloved hands would explore the cupboards for swabs, test tubes and culture dishes. Pretending to be a doctor, I would delight in swabbing my nose, mouth and ears, before rubbing the cotton samples across the surface of agar jelly on the petri dishes and placing them in the fridge.

I loved the anticipation of waiting for Dad to bring the petri dishes home weeks later, to see what had grown on the dishes. The only forbidden piece of equipment in the laboratory was the Bunsen burner, although I gave that my best try!

It felt like Dad changed overnight. In reality, it was more of a gradual change and we became more emotionally distant throughout 1981.

Dad had been the focus of my universe, but now had been replaced by an angry, unfamiliar figure. In physical form, he was still my dad, adored by many. He was the nucleus of his social circle and admired by his colleagues. At home, the reality was different, and our once strong inseparable connection hung by a thread.

The transformation left me confused, hurt and anxious. I spent many heart wrenching hours trying to work out what had happened. Suddenly, where there had once been love, hugs and kisses, now there was shouting and unexpected outbursts of anger, often directed at me.

Dad had always had a temper, a bit of a short fuse. You could say he was highly strung and a little anxious, but prior to that summer, his anger had always been towards other people. That's what made it so confusing.

That summer marked the beginning of my living as if walking on eggshells. I never knew when he would fly off the handle. Swipes to the head, arms and legs became commonplace and would come out of nowhere.

Small things would trigger an outburst. Like when I wanted to eat something different for supper, or go to bed later. Whatever the trigger, seconds before a strike, Dad would appear agitated. His face would flush a deep cherry red; his lips would purse; and his hands, shake.

It was upsetting and confusing. I found myself loving and hating Dad at the same time. I tried to retaliate, and would scream at him. The more I screamed, the more he screamed back. It became a chicken and egg situation.

I wasn't the easiest teenager. Truth be told, I tended to be highly strung and a little anxious myself. I didn't suffer fools, and I took no prisoners. It was the perfect storm.

Mum attempted to rationalise our new family dynamic, saying it was common in families. "Girls grow up and don't need their dads anymore," she had said after reading an article about parent-teenage friction in *Family Circle* magazine. "Don't provoke him Elizabeth," she pleaded, her eyes hopeful, sad, and desperate.

It never got any easier, though. By 1983, we couldn't enjoy a family dinner without a row. We were civil to each other in social situations and when we were with grandparents and other extended family, but behind closed doors, it was a battle ground.

In November 1983, when I was fifteen, I started two weeks' work experience at a car breakdown company, not far from where we lived. I felt grown up and confident on my first day. I walked into the office in a new Chelsea Girl outfit. I had a wonderful first day and felt so grown-up.

I was on such a high and wanted to share every detail with Mum and Dad over supper that evening. As it often did, the atmosphere at the dinner table felt tense and I didn't feel that a detailed account of my day would be welcome or appreciated. Feeling anxious, and in need of some space, I excused myself, having eaten only half of the cottage pie and vegetables on my plate. I said I was tired and wanted to get an early night to feel fresh for work the next day.

As I made my way upstairs, I was conscious that Dad was just behind me. I assumed he was going to use the bathroom upstairs as we only had one toilet in the house. I was on the sixth stair when I felt the swipe. It landed hard on the back of my head, jolting me forwards onto my knees. I was shocked and disorientated as I buried my crumpled face in my hands on top of the next stair.

The coarse weave of the carpet felt rough on my hands and knees. Within seconds, there were loud disapproving comments about my early departure from the dinner table and my dismissive attitude.

His accusations filled me with an instant incandescent rage. My body shook from head to toe. My eyes filled with angry tears. I turned round to face him, sobbing uncontrollably.

There was a look of resentment and exasperation on his flushed face and I could see his hands were shaking. "That's it," I screamed, "I am leaving this house, and I am reporting you" I said, as I pushed myself past him.

As I ran down the stairs, I was conscious that Mum and Jane were standing in the lounge doorway watching me. They were silent, their faces solemn. Their eyes pleaded with me not to leave.

But it was too late. Enough was enough. I grabbed my shoes, coat and purse and slammed the front door behind me. I ran down the road, choking on my tears, phone box in my sights, a ten pence coin at the ready in my tight fist. I dialled Childline, having kept the number hidden for months in the inside pocket of my purse. Two rings were followed by a gentle male voice. "Hello, can I help?"

"Sorry, I dialled the wrong number," I stammered, after a long pause.

Of course I couldn't report him, I loved him.

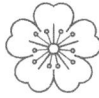

Chapter 4

You Are What You Think

I can't remember whether I gave up on school, or whether school gave up on me. It was probably a bit of both!

Around the age of thirteen, I thought my falling grades were driven by the fact I couldn't see the blackboard clearly. A trip to the opticians resulted in a pair of rather ugly blue-framed National Health Service glasses for my myopic eyes.

They fixed the physical issue, but I was still left feeling not good enough. There was pressure at home and endless hours of tense evening tuition at the dining room table with Dad; a last-ditch attempt to fix my fear of geometry, algebra and fractions. He was a natural at maths, hence the home tutoring, but with our relationship being as fractured as it was, the sessions were torturous. The pressure to be 'better' felt constant and exhausting.

I excelled at English, geography and biology, whilst Jane's talents lay in art. However, Dad made it crystal clear to both of us that university would be a no-go without a pass in maths.

By fourteen, with a string of non-memorable maths teachers behind me, I stopped caring. *It will be what it will be,*

I thought. There were more important things to think about anyway, in the order of fashion, discos and boys.

I adored fashion. As a young girl, I had accessories to match every outfit. Hair accessories, earrings, necklaces, rings, brooches, handbags, and even colour-coordinated bows for my shoes. I had the eye of a magpie for anything that shone. From a very young age, fashion gave me a sense of control in my life that I liked the feel of. I would pore over mum's clothes catalogues for hours, and find any opportunity to sneak into her wardrobes and try on her many outfits.

As soon as I was old enough to buy my own clothes, I would spend Saturdays with my best friend Ann looking through the racks of clothes in Chelsea Girl and Top Shop. We had to look just right for the weekly disco in our small, suburban town. 'Dress to impress,' was our motto and we took it seriously. We were the best dressed duo in our town. We loved every bit of the attention it brought us.

"You are what you wear," I used to say to Mum – my way of encouraging her to give me money for my weekly shopping trips. Bless her sweet soul, she usually did, and often without a word of disapproval. She knew shopping made me happy. The more I spent, the better I would feel, the more confident, the more in control; more like the girl I wanted to be. Bottom line: clothes made me feel good, they gave me my identity, they gave me my status.

What I didn't see then was that the clothes and sparkly bling may have looked beautiful on the outside, but my real beauty was lying underneath, within me. I had no idea I was *enough*, just as I was.

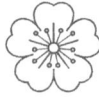

Chapter 5

Rebellion

May 1982. Confirmation day.

The day I would remember forever, according to my over-excited mum. The house was scrubbed from top to bottom. Externally beautiful.

The chlorine smell stuck in my throat and nostrils. The hoover had been out since 6.30 am and pine fragrance wood polish brought a shine to all the wooden surfaces. The house had to look pristine, a solid family home, happy and warm, comfortable, yet classy. That's the way Mum wanted others to see it.

I never saw it that way! Comfortable – yes, warm – yes, on a good day. On a bad day, my cherished miniature Whimsy animal collection floated like tiny rafts on my bedroom windowsill filled with melted water after a heavy night's frost.

"Appearances are everything," Mum used to say, and everything had to be just so. The energy in the house felt heavy and false that morning.

I sat up in bed, and noticed an unattractive reddish-purple

stain on the white cotton pillowcase. A smile broke across my sleepy face as I remembered I had died my hair the previous evening. I had rubbed crude food colouring from my scalp through to the ends of my edgy, Human League haircut.

I had no sense that it might go wrong. My school friends had used this method for months, creating some wonderful rich chestnut tones. I had been optimistic the night before. On seeing the stain, I felt a sense of foreboding. I wanted to avoid the mirror. I lay in bed for another ten minutes. Snuggled into the comfort and security of my soft Dorma duvet, I must have fallen asleep again.

I was awoken by a vivid dream. In my dream, I was standing in my pyjamas in the hallway, my Confirmation guests stood pointing at my hair with horrified faces. With that shocking image, I jolted awake, rubbed my weary eyes, and decided it was time to face the truth!

I stumbled towards the bathroom and stood in front of the large rectangular mirror above the white basin. It didn't look too bad, but not great either. It had more of a purple hue than the warm, burnt orange, autumnal look I had hoped for…

Mum walked in and pretended not to notice, but I sensed her disappointment. She diverted her gaze to the large plastic suit cover in her outstretched arms. "Well, darling, I've picked out something lovely for you to wear. It's a striking colour and it will match your hair. It's Laura Ashley." She smiled, and unzipped the cover. She took out an enormous puff ball of a dress, in dark mauve, with a smocked bodice and giant sleeves.

"I am not wearing that," I shouted, "it's hideous."

Calmly, she laid it down on the bed. "This is not open

for discussion, darling. We want you to look respectable and ladylike in church today. We want you to be the perfect Christian and goddaughter, so please get dressed and be ready to welcome everyone downstairs. They will be here soon."

My tongue pressed hard against the roof of my mouth and my eyes burned as I stood there, arms crossed, head bowed. I hated the day and what was expected of me. It wasn't me and neither was the dress.

One hour later, the guests started to pour in. It wasn't long before our neat hallway was full. Godmothers, godfathers, grandparents, aunts and uncles. All smiling. All looking for the star of the show, carrying their gifts: pendants, bibles, and photograph frames.

To my disappointment, there wasn't a blingy gift in sight!

"Oh, I'm so sorry," Mum said to one of my godmothers when I didn't say thank you. "We are in that stage, you know the one, the rebellious teen one."

"She'll come round," my godmother replied, a sympathetic, knowing smile, on her face. They both seemed oblivious to the fact I was standing right there.

Four hours, I told myself. *Just four hours*. I put on a smile.

I will endure this dog and pony show, then I will wash out my hair; it will have served its purpose.

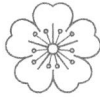

Chapter 6

Which Path?

School results day came and went.

What did I expect? To be honest, not much more than I got: a handful of good O-levels and I even scraped a pass for maths.

The grades would have secured a place at college to study A-levels. I knew that at some point, I wanted to be a doctor, but not yet. Right now, I wanted my independence and needed financial freedom to move out of the family home. I wanted a car, a flat and a job that paid well.

My wishes were very specific. The car had to be a red Alpha Romeo, which Dad said was another handbag on wheels!

I didn't have any idea of living costs and zero understanding of the declining job market in the early 1980s. At best, without A-levels, I was looking at a Youth Training Scheme in our local Halifax Building Society, earning just £25 per week. That wouldn't even keep my dream car running.

If I did A-levels, I would need to stay at home for another

two years and that was out of the question. Things were too tough with Dad. I was caught between a rock and a hard place. The reality felt grim. My options were limited, and I felt trapped.

It turned out I didn't have long to think about it. Within a fortnight, an application form had been laid out on the dining room table. Mum and Dad hovered over me with a fountain pen, a large manilla envelope and a first-class stamp. "It is the right thing to do," they both said, attempting to sound encouraging.

I groaned with boredom and despair. I didn't want to train to be a medical secretary. It wasn't my plan, and it wasn't me – I knew that for sure.

This wasn't my destiny. It was their plan. They felt it was a fair compromise because it was a college course, with a qualification upon completion, and a better option than the Youth Training Scheme. They thought the medical element would appeal to me, which, to be fair, it did, but I'd wanted to be a doctor, not a medical secretary. Even the school careers' adviser had shown his frustration, rolling his eyes at my unrealistic dreams, as he described them.

I dropped the large brown envelope, containing the completed form, into the postbox with a heavy heart. The dreams I had for my future were bobbing away on an inflatable lilo, destined to be beaten up by wild waves and lost forever in the ocean. Was this really my life? It felt small…

It took a week for the acceptance letter to arrive. Mum and Dad were overjoyed I was going to college. That was their narrative all along, even if it was to learn a job I had no interest in. I felt more trapped than ever, knowing there was no hope of me leaving home, now that I had a college place.

I never fitted in on the course. It felt too serious. To bring some humour and mischief to the class, I became disruptive. I would tell the girls exaggerated stories about my teenage exploits and sexual experimenting, with the intention of shocking and generating some banter in class.

My spirited antics kept me amused on a course that was attended by twelve young women who acted more like they were at a Swiss finishing school than a secretarial course. Many of them would arrive at college each day, proud as pea-cocks in their frilly blouses, tucked into sharp pencil skirts, shorthand pads at the ready. Quite the opposite to my casual denims, Converse pumps and carefree demeanour. "Why fit in, when you can stand out?" I used to say to Mum as I left for college each morning. She knew I wasn't happy and would shake her head in despair.

Two years later, I left with a Diploma in Medical Secretarial Studies.

Despite my rebellious mischief, I was the first to secure a full-time medical secretarial role in a local hospital.

I talked my way into the job interview. I met a friendly chap in a local night club who held the position of Head of Medical Records at the hospital. He told me about this vacancy for a medical secretary in the orthopaedic department. Much to his astonishment, I strolled into the hospital the next day and asked for him by name at reception. The look on his face had been a picture! I left the hospital thirty minutes later with an interview scheduled for the following week.

One week later, I had my first job offer. It was not the job I wanted – not the job I felt in my heart I was destined to do, but I was on the career ladder.

On the positive side, I was earning money, running a car and looking for a flat. I had made that happen. I had seen the opportunity and grabbed it. Perhaps I had more control over my life than I thought?

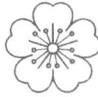

Chapter 7

Young Love, First Love

You know when you know…

That's what people say about relationships. That was certainly my experience when I laid eyes on my first love, aged sixteen.

He was in a phone box at the time which I was waiting to use. I have always trusted my gut feel. It wasn't the most romantic proposition, but my inner knowing told me it felt right. Our flirtatious eyes locked and I knew we would be an item. His eyes, a deep blue, almost navy, slightly rounded, and partially covered by a mop of thick sandy brown hair; my eyes, a bluey green, almond in shape, framed by a blonde bob with a sharp fringe.

I wouldn't say I felt fireworks, but there was an inevitability to our attraction and connection.

I had been out with quite a few other boys. There had been a procession of colourful characters, as my parents used to call them. They were the ones I had deliberately dated, and invited back to the family home, with the sole intention to shock!

They didn't have to impress anyone in our family as I wasn't serious about them, but the boyfriends I did care about weren't always a suitable choice for our family either. There were so many hoops for them to jump through. Some of them complained they had been subjected to an interview when they first entered our home, as opposed to a relaxed chat over supper. Dad said I needed to date someone with good credentials – a high academic achiever from a middle-class family with a professional career.

"A guy with enough money to keep you in good clothes and handbags," he used to say.

I could keep myself in good clothes and handbags, thank you very much!

The date with my first love didn't start well, though.

We had agreed to meet at a wine bar and he was late because the traffic had been heavy getting into the city. His dad had driven him in, and I chose to take the bus on what I thought would be a warm July evening, only to be caught in an unexpected downpour.

I had paid special attention to my outfit. I'd paired my white bermuda shorts with my favourite white stiletto shoes. In the rain, my fake tan had stained my shorts and run down my legs. The orange streaks looked awful.

My face flushed with humiliation as I attempted to greet my date with a cheerful smile and a flick of my crimped, bobbed hair. To calm my nerves, I drank too many cherry Bs, which went straight to my head, and I ended up spilling one down the front of my yellow T-shirt. It was not an attractive sight!

He had dressed up, wearing a pair of narrow fit beige

chinos, a short-sleeved white shirt and a skinny dark blue necktie, which was loosely tied. I thought the tie looked out of place against the chinos, but who was I to criticise in my orange shorts and stained T-shirt?!

The conversation flowed well and there were no awkward silences. We giggled and flirted, and the hours passed quickly. There was a goodnight kiss, with an invitation to a second date, which led to a third and a fourth, before I lost count.

We were always together. Of course, family approval had to be sought, and there were the usual questions about family background, academic achievement and career prospects.

With those boxes ticked; months turned into years. Before we knew it, we had been going steady for five years. There were many twists and turns in our relationship over the years. We loved each other but there were regular break-ups and make-ups. We were young, childhood sweethearts, and nothing seemed to keep us apart for long. We were given the accolade of being named the Liz Taylor and Richard Burton of our small town.

It was simple at the beginning.

We were discovering ourselves, attempting to find our direction in life.

Neither of us had much, but we both had dreams and spirit.

It mattered what people thought of us and appearances were everything.

We were strong and popular characters within our friendship circle.

We were each a bit lost.

Who knew we would end up being together for thirty years?!

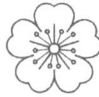

Chapter 8

A New City

"You are moving where?" Dad shouted.

It was a wet mid-summer morning in 1990.

"Plymouth in Devon," I said, my voice unwavering. I made direct eye contact and forced a smile.

"Yes, I know exactly where it is," Dad replied. "My question is; why on earth would you want to move there? It is a naval fishing town. There are no job prospects, and you will end up packing fish."

The move wasn't up for debate – not through my lens anyway. I had made up my mind weeks ago. I had even put a deposit down on an apartment rental. My boyfriend had secured a place to study at Plymouth University and after five years of going strong, I was going with him and that was that. Decision made. I instinctively knew it was the right thing to do.

The next eight weeks dragged. Dad's pessimistic gloom around my future career opportunities plummeted by the day. In contrast, I was excited. I was going somewhere far away, to make a new life in a different city for three whole years. I would make new friends, enjoy new experiences, and even if that did mean packing fish for a living, so be it!

Moving day saw my beloved red Alpha Romeo packed to the gunnels. I insisted on taking every item in my wardrobe, including my large handbag and shoe collection. In addition to my clothes and accessories, Mum's oldest saucepans, a kettle, an iron and a toasted sandwich maker all made the final cut into my crammed boot.

We made it feel like home quickly.

I was so happy, other than shedding a few tears when Mum telephoned to make sure we had arrived safely.

I was doing OK until I heard her voice. I felt a deep sense of guilt that I had left her. She sounded so forlorn and was clearly missing me already.

I struggled to dismiss the thought, saying out loud to myself: *This is my time.*

I set to work, hoovering and polishing each room, scrubbing clean the damp and cracking magnolia walls. We went to Ikea on a mission to find cheap soft furnishings to brighten the place up. I hung pictures and laid rugs around the spacious living area and arranged artificial flowers in little stained-glass vases. I intended to stamp our identity onto this modest first home.

The furnishings that came with the apartment appeared to be high quality, most of them Laura Ashley. There was a heavy smell of wood because most of the furniture was pine or oak. Each piece seemed blocky in appearance – too large for the space it occupied. In fact, with all the wood, the apartment looked an orange shade of brown, overlaid with red, green and cream soft furnishings.

Love it, or hate it, we had to live with it as we couldn't afford to change it. I was the only one earning money and I hadn't found a job yet. Five days later, that all changed, when I was offered a job at the local hospital. So much for fish packing!

In my search for work, I chose to cover all the city hospitals on foot. It felt like the right thing to do. Trusting my gut, and equipped with my CV, references and a kickass attitude, I set out early.

As I approached the first hospital, I felt a little nervous. I decided to take a moment outside, to consider my introduction.

Whenever I felt anxious in life, my remedy had aways been to talk out loud to myself. It usually worked. *Just put on your big girl pants Lizzie, smile sweetly, and ask the question,* I said to myself.

Do you have any vacancies for an excellent medical secretary? That approach had worked before. Why wouldn't it again?

Sure enough, I hit the jackpot on day two, hospital number three, of my walk-in strategy. I had an interview two days later which resulted in a job offer, with a start date for the following Monday.

I was going to work as a medical secretary for a consultant urologist, who specialised in male erectile disorders.

Life just kept getting better!

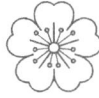

Chapter 9

Different faces, Different days

By now, I was in my early twenties, and I'd started to build a new life in a new city.

My mindset also started to change. I don't remember how it started, or whether the change was in my head, heart, or both, but something felt very different. Some days I would feel really confident and carefree, my natural extroverted nature making me visible and larger-than-life. On other days, I could be as quiet as a church mouse, and all I wanted to do was hide away in a corner.

I was carrying the guilt of leaving Mum behind. I loved her so much and knew that deep down, she wasn't happy, but she seemed to have a way of blocking anything painful out of her mind, focusing only on the things that made her life look full and perfect to herself and others. I knew that was her survival tool and it served her well. I respected that, and although my ego wanted to save her, my inner wisdom knew she had to save herself. She had made her own life choices. There had been opportunities for her to take a different path, but she always remained stoic and loyal with her 'marriage is for life' ethos. I knew I had to leave her to get on with her life, just as I had to get on with mine.

I was making friends, but there were days when I felt detached, like I was observing my life through a window. In my eyes, nothing I did seemed to be quite enough to meet the high expectations I put on myself.

Had I made enough friends? Did I have a good work life balance? Were we entertaining as much as we should? Was I earning enough money? And so, the list went on!...

Perfection was expected and I was conditioned to be my harshest critic. It took up so much energy. At that point in my life, I hadn't realised I didn't have to pay attention to that conditioned thinking. I was more than enough just as I was.

The truth is, I was living on my nerves. I was anxious and could feel very up or very down. I didn't feel like I fitted in and I worried about whether I was liked by others. I wanted to be a confident and independent woman. Some days I did feel those things; but on other days, I wanted to blend into the background.

I would hear my friends say I was capable of pretty much anything I set my mind to. There were times when it suited me to show up with this hard-faced, get-on-with-it persona. On those days, I would find myself getting irritated with others' indecisiveness. I would make knee-jerk judgements, my frustration evident on my face and in my tone. But my biggest judgements were always directed at myself – self-kindness was out of the question.

On other days, I was the exact opposite.

There was no judgement of myself or others.

I loved the world, I was full of empathy, kindness and compassion.

I was analysing and worrying about everything during that period of life readjustment.

It was confusing, inconsistent, and draining.

In our first year of living together, I felt so overwhelmed that I decided to take a rare trip back home for the Easter holiday weekend. I had plucked up the courage to have an honest conversation with Mum about my feelings. I was unsure how to kick off the chat, so I asked her outright how she would describe me as a person.

She looked surprised at the question, and, for a moment, I didn't think she was going to answer. She stopped washing up and gazed out of the kitchen window. When she replied, her words were unexpected, and at the same time, intriguing.

"Capable, tough, a little hard, but kind underneath," she said, and then, after a thoughtful pause: "Dad and I are very proud of you, and we love you very much."

I wanted to question the description, but I didn't. I couldn't.

I couldn't find the right words to challenge her description.

My mind raced, and I wondered who I really was. Did Mum know me? The real me? Did she know I was hurting inside? I felt like a tangled ball of wool. Perhaps I was capable, tough and hard.

There are benefits to being those things in life – they had served me well over the years. Each one of those attributes had played its part in helping me build a protective wall around myself as my relationship with Dad had broken down. In my childhood innocence, that was the only way I saw to survive.

I had survived, and now I was free. I didn't need that wall anymore. I could relax, let go, but old habits die hard. Even though I was living in my own apartment, two hundred miles from my family home, my emotional scars hadn't healed and my fighting spirit was undeterred. I saw no inner beauty in myself – only damage.

As the days and months followed, my questions only grew…

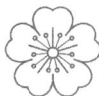

Chapter 10

A Turning Point

When I am ready for something, be it a task or a challenge, I am ready! If appropriate, I will communicate my decision, take the relevant action, and usually succeed.

When I jump before I am ready, or when I am not certain about something, or my heart isn't in it, then I don't always succeed. It's as simple as that, really. My philosophy: *When you know, you know!*

On my twenty-fourth birthday, I was ready. I announced to family and friends that I was going back to college to complete three A-levels so I could secure a place at university.

The response to my announcement was mixed. Many of my friends were both surprised and supportive in equal measure. My boyfriend was delighted. My sister said, "Go for it, Sis." Mum said she was proud.

Dad said I had missed the boat and was too old, making the point that it was not a practical, thought-through decision. My boyfriend's parents had similar concerns: "Why don't you two just settle down? Keep steady jobs, buy a semi, have a couple of kids, enjoy a holiday in Spain every year?" Then the jaw dropper, "Why not just be normal? You're nothing special, you know!"

I couldn't, for the life of me, understand why it was such a big deal to them. I wasn't asking for money to fund the venture, or even a place to live. Bottom line: I was hungry to learn, striving to improve my education, eager to build my life, with the opportunity to experience new realities in the process.

How was that a problem?

I had wasted more than enough time already. I didn't like blowing my own trumpet, but I knew I was bright and more than capable of securing a place at university.

I don't think anyone expected my plan. It wasn't in their narrative for my future, so they didn't expect it to be in mine. Their cynicism and scepticism only served to fuel my energy, as I conducted my research with gusto.

I made it my top priority to create my own destiny.

Energised, I researched colleges and university degree courses in my favourite subjects: psychology and biology. Whilst on this mission, I came across an opportunity to apply for a summer camp counsellor position in the USA. I had found the vacancy on a college notice board. I figured that, if successful, I would meet like-minded people at camp, who were either already on degree courses, or about to start them. It seemed like a good way forward as it would be a year before I could start college. I had read somewhere that if you surround yourself with people who inspire you, you are more likely to fulfil your personal ambitions.

I applied for a place. If I got a position, it would give me just under a year in the States, so I could go backpacking after the summer camp season had finished. I was ready to see as much of the country as possible before I started the one-year condensed A-level courses, which would secure my university place for the following academic year.

The summer camp interview was a breeze. They loved me and I loved them. Before I could change my mind, I found myself at Heathrow Airport, with a rucksack on my back and my passport and plane ticket gripped in my palm. *This is just the start*, I sang to myself, as I raced towards my boarding gate, ponytail protruding from my red and blue Camp America baseball cap.

Tucked away, high in the wild Adirondack Mountains of upstate New York, I experienced complete clarity of thought, acceptance of who I was, and a realisation of what I needed to do in my life. It would be easy to say that it was the stunning surroundings that triggered my clear thinking, but I knew that the shift was coming from within me. The mountain air might well have been purer, but so were my thoughts. I had been holding on too tightly, and I had allowed myself to let go.

There was something magical about the camp that has never left my memory. The neat little rows of brightly painted wooden cabins, a quirky door knocker, with a number on each one. The hard metal-framed bunk beds with their crisp white sheets and thick brown blankets. The alluring wide lake, with its crystal-clear water, which always shimmered, whatever the weather, framed by scenic mountains and tall forest firs.

I can still hear the peals of laughter ringing out from the tiny cabins from as early as 6 am. Each day brought its own crazy routine, underpinned by an unconditional love and the simplicity of an unmaterialistic, non-judgmental environment.

It felt truthful, untarnished, and structured.

We ate together. We played games, sang, and danced together.

At the end of each action-packed day, we bunked down in our cozy cabins.

Camp felt safe, like a happy family.

I adored it. I was home.

The time there passed way too quickly.

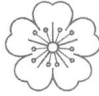

Chapter 11

A New Reality

At university, I soon realised the more effort you put in, the more you got out. That went for coursework grades, as well as fun!

Before arriving, I made a decision not to share my age with anyone. I had always looked younger than my years and was more baby-faced than most of my peers, so it wasn't a surprise when the young crowd took me under their wing. They might have suspected I was a little older, but they weren't phased by it, and neither was I.

I was having the time of my life, settling into my basic but comfortable hall of residence. I registered for clubs, rock climbing, and water skiing, and partied in the student union and nightclubs with an energy I had never experienced before.

I enjoyed the financial challenge of building an edgy, but flattering, student wardrobe. It was a blast. I had it well sussed out that if I got ahead and wrote my essays early, I would not only get the best pick of the books and journals in the library, but I would also be free to party when others had to work all night to ensure they submitted their work on time.

Being able to type made the essay process a lot easier and saved me hours in front of the computer. My working methods made me a secret swot, but no one needed to know that. I felt in complete control of my workload, which had to be balanced with my two part-time jobs – a necessity to pay my bills and rent.

Working and studying was a juggling act and required huge self-discipline. One of the jobs was medical secretarial work, which I was a dab hand at, but it did involve working overnight several times a week, audio typing for hours in dimly-lit hospital offices.

The other job was a little more controversial, but had shorter hours, and the money kept me in good shoes: I was an Ann Summers Party Planner. Even with two jobs, to my surprise and delight, I was a consistent grade A student. Who would have known? Certainly not me!

Despite my dreams and outward appearance, and all my assertions to the contrary, I had still worried that my dad was right when he said I would never achieve much.

Three years passed quickly. Before I knew it, I was gowned and marching with pride across the polished parquet floor towards the stage in the grand university hall. I had achieved a BSc Honours degree in Human Psychology. I couldn't stop smiling.

Mum and Dad attended, of course. They clapped with enthusiasm and took lots of photographs, both proud and delighted by my achievement. It was a wonderful day, and my face glowed with delight and fulfilment. There was no reference to previous concerns around my academic ability, or the fact that I had missed the boat!

As I flopped down, exhausted, on top of my soft duvet that warm July evening, I had an insight that came and went in a flash: I had done it. I had exceeded my own – and others' – expectations of me. Any tiny doubts that I might have had about my abilities had been proved wrong. I didn't have to pay them any attention now. I hoped that was the end of them.

They didn't stop, but I stopped listening to them. That's when my career finally took off.

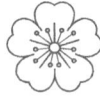

Chapter 12

The Corporate Ladder

I expected to feel different after I got my degree. That bit of paper was supposed to make me feel powerful and relevant in the world, capable of anything – the ability to hold my own in challenging discussions and situations, to articulate myself in a clear and confident manner. I expected it to give me a competitive edge, to make me feel whole – as good as everyone else.

I felt no different from how I did before, and now I was at a crossroads in my life. There was an opportunity to stay at university and do a PhD in criminal or clinical psychology. There was also a university that had welcomed my application to study medicine as a mature graduate.

While these offers were tempting, I was self-funding, and money was tight. It felt like the right time to find a job. This time, I used my medical secretarial connections and secured a graduate role in the pharmaceutical industry as a medical sales representative. This played to my passion for anything medical, yet sometimes I felt I had sold myself short in terms of applying my psychology degree or training to be a doctor.

Me being me, though, I was determined to make the best of my new opportunity and worked hard to prove myself.

To sell medical products, the most important part of the job was making connections and building relationships with medical professionals in general practice and hospitals. I surprised myself at how I took to sales. It was scary at first, but once I got to know my customers and understood what they needed, it was quite easy and had many perks. I had a flashy sports car and enjoyed more than generous pay cheques.

It wasn't long before I had paid off my student loans and we could put a deposit down on our first house, a tiny end-of-terrace Victorian which we thought was a palace. It was a narrow red brick property with a huge bay window at the front. The bottle green front door opened into a cozy lounge with original features, including a tiled antique fireplace.

The only problem was the slugs! There were many deep cracks in the wooden panelling under the sash bay in the lounge. After a wet night, we would come downstairs to find silvery slug trails glistening across the maroon carpet - not the most welcoming sight first thing in the morning!

The house was modest, but at the age of twenty-nine, we had a mortgage, two steady jobs, two cars, and we were still going strong, despite our travelling and our breakups and makeups.

Those early years were good. We had sacrificed so much for so long. It was a treat to have regular money, and it felt like we were back in the honeymoon phase of our relationship. We enjoyed socialising, had regular meals out, booked holidays abroad, and visited friends across the UK. Life was good, but underneath, I had the nagging feeling that we were heading for a fall…

We both worked in the same industry, for a start, which I didn't consider to be healthy. Neither of us could say no to a party invitation, whether that be a joint invitation or a solo one. Sometimes, instead of being on the same side, it felt like we were in competition. We were both working in sales across a similar geographic territory, which, in itself, created a new dynamic.

Our social circle grew, but I wasn't keen on some of his new work friends, which created tension, as I would often decline invitations to socialise with them and their girlfriends. I preferred to see our original friends.

I put the hours in, keen for early promotion to a management role, but he soon became underwhelmed with the industry and resented the time and energy I devoted to my job, which often took me away from home for days at a time.

At my first company sales conference in Athens, I was offered a glimpse into what might lie ahead. I ignored it at the time.

I was excited about the conference. I had never been to one before. It sounded so glamorous. It was a great excuse for me to buy lots of new clothes and meet new people.

It's funny how things never turn out how you expect them to. With such high expectations, I was left feeling disappointed. I had packed a wardrobe for the anticipated warmth of Athens in May, but it rained the whole time. I thought I'd get to see the city, but we were booked into a hotel miles away from the city centre.

The hotel was large, concrete and soulless. There were no windows in the business rooms and little natural air anywhere. The air conditioning system was fierce and loud. I shivered in my new short-sleeved, cream linen trouser suit, goose bumps visible on my spray-tanned forearms.

During the black-tie awards dinner on the second night, a colleague said to me, "You look so happy and excited about everything, it has to be your first job in the industry?"

"Yes," I replied, smiling at him.

"Wait until you have been around thirty years – it isn't as much fun then," he said with a gloomy expression.

"Why?" I asked, my face innocent, wondering why I had been seated next to the oldest person in the sales team.

When he answered, he had tears in his eyes. "It will change you. It will take, and keep on taking, from you."

I didn't know how to reply to that, so I said, "Oh, that doesn't sound very good. I hope I will never feel that way. Why do you stay if you don't like it?"

His reply was short. I sensed he wanted to end the conversation. He appeared restless as he fidgeted with his table napkin.

"It's the golden handcuffs," he said. "It buys you. It has bought me. Now I can't leave. I have too much to lose. I am trapped."

I wasn't going to let him deter me, so I ended the conversation, heading off to find someone more positive to talk to. Despite the bounce in my step, I had a feeling there was a tsunami on its way, headed right in my direction.

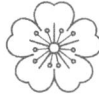

Chapter 13

What's not to love

It was January 2002, and we had moved from our old Victorian terraced house into a four-bedroom detached new-build.

We had packed our belongings in an orderly fashion into large brown boxes, taped them up and labelled them with black marker pen. I stared out of the curtainless bedroom window, my expression blank. I took in the scene outside our picture book house, with its neat flagstone path and turfed lawn.

My future mother-in-law stood next to me. "What next?" she asked, her tone enthusiastic and excited. "Do we hear wedding bells, the patter of tiny feet? You have everything now: a great job, a beautiful home. It's not like that for everyone; I can tell you. You are lucky, Liz. You have made it."

Whilst her words sounded complimentary, I felt like she thought I was ungrateful – that I took my life for granted.

"Made what?" I answered.

"Your life, its perfect" she said.

I wanted to smile. I wanted to say, *I know, I am excited*, but the words wouldn't come out of my mouth. I stuttered and avoided her deep stare.

"Oh right, I know," I stammered. I felt like she could see straight into my soul. I suspected she could sense I was losing my way.

"I'm not ok, not really. I feel like something is missing. I feel so low some days. I pretend it's all OK, but it's not. I shop a lot. We see friends. We travel to nice places. It helps, but only for a little while, and then I get low again."

Her disdainful grey eyes ran over me, from the top of my head to the toes on my feet. "You have everything you could ever want. I had nothing at your age. You don't know how lucky you are."

I lowered my head towards the floor. My eyes welled up with tears of embarrassment.

"You might think I have everything, but I don't feel like I'm myself anymore. The real me got lost somewhere a long time ago, and I can't get it back."

She continued to glare at me, while her eyes – dark and sharp as a laser, delved for an answer.

I felt exposed. I stared at the cream twist pile bedroom carpet, the flecks of gold, turquoise and pink. Bits of fluff lined the room where the fitter's knife had hacked away at the edges of the carpet.

She took my hand with a firm grasp, squeezing my fingers so hard they felt crushed against my rings. "It's life. Just plain old simple life. This is your lot. Be grateful. Get on with it," she said. "I'll make us a cup of tea."

Her tone was haunting. Her smile didn't meet her eyes.

She dropped my hand like it was a hot coal and walked out.

I stood there, speechless, rigid, angry, vulnerable. *You idiot*, I thought to myself. Why had I shared my deepest feelings with her? I thought she might understand.

By the time I had turned around, she was back, unpacking boxes and arranging the furniture. My life was being organised right in front of my eyes. I felt exhausted and powerless.

I took a deep breath, threw back my head, flicked out my hair and forced the corners of my mouth to turn up. I'd stepped into my protective shield, the familiar heavy coat of armour. I felt its comfort, protection and power.

"Champagne is in order," I said. "Let's celebrate our beautiful home and perfect life."

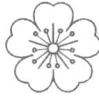

Chapter 14

Trappings

Of course, we tied the knot. It had always been the plan. We were childhood sweethearts and cared about each other.

The pressure from our parents to make it official had been immense. In the end, we got married on a beach, far away, on our own, without telling a soul. Whilst our parents were delighted to hear our news when we returned home, they were not happy that they hadn't been involved in our big day.

It was a magical wedding, and I have no regrets. When I made my vows, I meant every word and wanted them to be for life. Sadly, the magic didn't last for many years after our special day.

I can't remember the exact day, month or year when our relationship started to break down. It was a long, slow death. The realisation was heartbreaking, particularly when I had known and loved him for most of my life.

Having once been best friends, we became strangers. Neither of us wanted to address it – we both chose to shirk away from the tough conversations. Our lives went in different directions. We lost our connection and seemed powerless to stop it. We were both unhappy, living in single cells of destructive isolation, which led to hours of loneliness and despair. There was a bitterness to our conversations that turned into toxic resentment and, eventually, a marital breakdown.

My vice was shopping. I shopped to forget, way beyond a healthy level, while he went to the pub. Both strategies served a purpose, and both were equally destructive. We stopped talking to each other.

Despite the strain, though, we kept going.

We tried our best to make it work. We went on fantastic holidays. American road trips were our thing. We had a mutual love of the open road and adored being spontaneous and making our seat-of-the-pants plans, as opposed to the rigid structure of more organised holidays.

There were blessings that came along too, like our beloved Jack Russell puppy who demanded, in her own doggy way, that we act like civilised grown-up parents, whatever the circumstances. She expected us to respond in united bliss to her every need and whimper. We did, of course! She was adorable – the baby we never had, and she will live in our hearts forever.

We joined a charity club in our local town. We treated everyone, including ourselves, to public displays of marital harmony every Tuesday night, whilst chatting through agenda items over a hot supper.

We were giving it our best shot, but it was getting harder and harder.

Over time, we started doing less and less together. Gone were the days when we might have enjoyed a weekend away together, or a long walk in the hills. Saturdays were now the day I would head into the city alone, to shop till I dropped, and he would head to the pub. Neither of us wanted to be home.

On we went, battling through each day for many years. We plastered over the cracks, remembered our history, indulged in fond teenage memories and happier days. We fooled everyone close to us. No one saw our misery or our pain. We pretended to be perfect, locked in happy memories, pretending to make more, but the scars were getting too deep to heal, and we were both exhausted from trying.

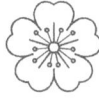

Chapter 15

Make or Break

It was make-or-break time. We needed something to reignite our relationship.

We had always been motivated by travel and exploring. The more adventure in a trip, the better. It was something we both had in common. Our nomadic spirits had fuelled our passion for backpacking holidays around the US, Europe and Southeast Asia.

There had been quite a few countries on our list to explore. My beautiful globe was one of my most treasured possessions. I would spin it around at least once a day, using a magnifying glass to zoom in on every detail, as I pondered what might be possible. This time, though, we weren't planning a backpacking adventure or a road trip. We had broken with our norm and booked a package holiday: a fortnight on the western coast of Mexico. The promise of deserted golden beaches, Mariachi bands, Pacific sunsets and a never-ending supply of tequila was intoxicating. We were both excited.

The venue was as breathtaking as the brochure and met every one of our expectations. On our second day, I said to myself, "If we can't have the time of our lives here, we really are broken."

With unlimited zest, we packed every minute of our days with activities. We explored the winding, cobbled streets of the old town, went horseback riding in the mountains, took a safari trip into the rain forest, did some whale watching, and were regulars at the beach barbeques each evening, with their never-ending supply of tequila and fajitas.

By the end of the first week, we were in a good place and quite exhausted. We made the decision to relax on the stunning beach for a few days.

Despite being an extrovert, I have never been a great fan of making friends on holiday. A bit of harmless small talk around the pool is fine, but I draw the line at much more than that. As I saw it, it wasn't anyone else's business what we did for a living, where we worked, how old we were and which room we were staying in.

Patty and Bud from Arizona appeared nice enough. A middle-aged couple with their own catering business, enjoying their time-share for a fortnight. They were taking a break from their teenage kids and demanding schedules.

Bud looked older than Patty, at a guess, late fifties. Patty looked around fiftyish. He was balding, slightly overweight, and his lime green Hawaiian shirt buttons strained around his bulbous belly, which hung over his long white shorts. She wore her thick grey hair in a long-plaited ponytail which almost reached the small of her back. She had a round face with a slightly ruddy complexion and wore baggy denim dungarees with black sequinned flip-flops.

They seemed harmless enough, almost parental, as they chatted with big smiles, asking us questions about our Mexican adventures so far. I didn't ask for doubles, but we got into rounds, and every time it was their turn to buy, my drink tasted extra strong, so I can only assume it was a double, or even a triple shot.

As the sun set and the evening turned into night, it wasn't a big surprise when they suggested we go out to dinner together. This was easy enough as their time-share complex was situated adjacent to our hotel, sharing the same bars and restaurants. We enjoyed a tasty traditional dinner, fajitas and enchiladas, washed down with some cheap local wine.

By eleven o'clock, I was ready to call it a night. We both were, but Patty and Bud were adamant that we should go and have a nightcap in their condo. Who were we to argue!?

As soon as we got through the door, I felt my spine tingle. I knew something was off. I couldn't put my finger on it, but their whole demeanour changed. No more nice chat, and suddenly there was nothing parental about them at all.

Bud wanted to show us around the condo. He dawdled at the hot tub on the balcony, saying, "My fox of a daughter likes to make out in here when she brings her boyfriends to stay."

Patty was being more tactile than she had been at the bar and restaurant, and had a different look in her eyes, which lingered a bit too long on the both of us. Bud asked us what we wanted to drink. Following my instincts, I declined. My husband asked for a Coke. I had no idea what he was thinking because there had been no opportunity to ask him. Patty and Bud hadn't left our side since they let us into the condo. I needed a wee but couldn't face the thought of heading to the toilet on my own. As far as I was concerned, the writing was on the wall: we had to get out of there; they clearly wanted a foursome.

Ten minutes, I told myself. Just ten minutes for him to drink his coke, and then we can thank them for their hospitality and leave. I nudged him and whispered, "Drink up quick, we need to go."

We sat down on the L-shaped sofa, both choosing to squeeze into the same corner of it. He swigged his drink and, to keep it natural, I asked Patty some questions about their condo and who had decorated it.

Generic conversation to neutralise the situation. I didn't really care; the décor was awful! After about five minutes, I stood up, saying we needed to go, but just as I said the words, my husband slumped forward like a sack of potatoes, his head hanging forward between his knees.

"What have you given him?" I said as they both sat and laughed at my emotional outburst. My face was flushed, and my skin was crawling with disgust and humiliation.

I dragged him off the sofa with every bit of strength I had. He was rambling, almost incoherent. I was charged, adrenaline in full flow. I don't know how I found the energy to drag him off that sofa and out of the condo, but I did.

The more I dragged his lifeless body, the more they laughed. Once out of their condo and in the elevator, I asked a friendly-looking young couple to help me. They were shocked by our story. We made it back to our hotel room.

I sat bolt upright, shaking for most of the night, trying to piece it all together while he lay in a deep sleep beside me. I checked his breathing at regular intervals throughout the night and was more than relieved when he awoke unscathed at 8 am the following morning. He remembered everything.

We played it safe that morning and stuck to the main hotel beach – no wandering off into the time-share grounds. But as we walked towards the sun loungers, we saw them: Patty and Bud headed straight in our direction.

I wanted to ignore them, but there was something inside me that wanted to call them out. In the cold light of day, in this public space, what could they do to us anyway? With that reassurance, I headed towards them and asked them what they had put in the glass of coke. As they answered, they looked straight into my accusing, angry eyes; theirs, cold and snake-like, "I'm sorry, Miss, do we know you?" It was ninety degrees Fahrenheit. A shiver ran up my spine…

I will never forget that holiday, and I count my blessings that we kept ourselves safe and survived to tell the tale. That holiday kept us going for a few more years. Like a band-aid covering a cut, it protected our wounds, patching us up as we continued to navigate life's twists and turns.

What I know now is that no holiday destination, however stunning, could repair what had already broken down within us.

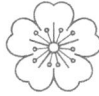

Chapter 16

Loyal, hopeless and lost

April 2011.

I looked in the mirror and hated what I saw. Staring back at me was a thin, nervous shell of a woman.

Prince William and Kate Middleton had just got married. They were so loved-up and gorgeous. I cried as I watched them take their vows on television. I was crying for them, and crying for me. I remembered the magic of my special day and how important our vows had been to both of us.

There were also tears for Dad, who had died just a few months before. In late 2009, he was diagnosed with cancer and became very sick. He died twelve months later, aged sixty-nine.

Dad and I had many challenges in our relationship over the years, but his death knocked me for six. I struggled to accept the finality of it. I had wanted to fix our relationship, and the sad thing is, I think he did too, but it never really got resolved. Even when we said our final goodbyes, it was like the words wouldn't come out of our mouths. Maybe they didn't need to be said. In his own way, I know he loved me. And in my own way, I loved him.

There were some tears over my uncertain future. Worst of all, I cried hard for the daily heartache that engulfed me about my marriage. As I watched the young lovers on screen, I feared, at forty-three, I would never feel happy again. My friends and colleagues saw multiple faces; whatever suited from day to day.

The grim reality was that my hands shook all the time, and I sat on them to control them. I was drinking too much wine and shopping too much because that blotted out my pain. In my mind, I had to show I was tough and resilient, a machine, capable of anything. If only they all knew. What a disaster!

Mum had started to ask questions. She seemed more curious and perceptive since she had become a widow. I would catch her looking at me, carefully observing my tiny frame and loose jeans. She had started to take bundles of washing from me and cook us the odd meal. I think she knew I was sinking. I wondered if she could see the pain behind my once-shining eyes.

To her credit, she kept drilling, but I kept clamming up. I felt locked in the chains of my own making as I stared at the television screen, my eyes like watery green ice.

What I knew, with certainty, was that I was about to hurt a lot of people in the quest to live my truth…

Leaving my marriage was the toughest thing I've ever done in my life so far. I had loved my husband for most of my life, since I was a teenager. It destroyed me emotionally and physically, yet I knew I had to do it. I looked in the mirror every morning and every evening for months, and talked to myself: *You must do this, Lizzie. You are going to have to be very grown-up and brave and leave this house and everything in it. There is no option; you must be selfish and be true to yourself.*

Every time I said those words, I felt a little bit stronger in my own skin. It was like I was giving myself a good talking to, yet self-soothing at the same time, keeping myself on the straight and narrow.

Although nothing prepared me for the day, I packed up a case and hold-all and announced I was leaving. It was heartbreaking for both of us. It would have been so easy to stay, to put up with everything, but I knew we were both worn out and worth so much more than that. We had more dignity and pride than that. We had more life to live.

I left in January 2013. It was time.

I knew it, and I didn't look back. I was afraid that if I did, I wouldn't have the courage to leave. My inner strength guided me that day as I remained calm, dignified and determined. As I shut the front door behind me, I kept my gaze ahead and my feet moving forward as I walked down our front path towards my car.

It was done.

I still deeply cared for my husband, but I had set us free, so we could both be the people we wanted to be.

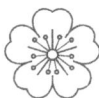

Chapter 17

Fresh Start

People often say that five of the most stressful things in a person's life are the death of a family member, illness, divorce, moving house and changing career. Well, there I was, aged forty-four, and trying to navigate four of those life events at the same time.

Yes, I was free, and given how unhappy I had been, that was a relief, but I was also grieving for everything, and everybody, I had lost in the process. I was trying to settle into a new town in the southeast of England, over a hundred miles away from where I had spent most of my life. Not only that, I had a new career as a business consultant, having been made redundant from the pharmaceutical industry a couple of years before. I felt like I was living in a dream and about to wake up at any moment. It was surreal…

The first few weeks were the worst. After a short stay with a girlfriend from work, which was functional, but not sustainable, I rented a small apartment. I was missing my dog and the familiarity of my old house, town and friends.

The apartment was modern and overlooked a busy canal. I would sit on the balcony for hours staring at the colourful barges passing by, and the never-ending stream of cyclists and dog walkers on the narrow tow path.

As tranquil as this scene might sound, the changes in my life had felt so intense and abrupt that I was overwhelmed – like a rabbit in the headlights. This emotional overwhelm consumed every ounce of my energy, to the point that I was finding it tough to get out of bed each morning and face the world, although I always did, of course.

I was determined to make the adjustment work and have never been known to change my mind once a decision is made, however uncomfortable the reality. The move had been my choice, but the truth was that every certainty in my life had been challenged, which left me feeling exposed, vulnerable and out of control.

I had a constant nervous feeling inside my tummy. I found it almost impossible to control my shaky hands. My weight was plummeting, and I had deep furrows on my brow. I waited for the feeling to pass, reassured by my friends and various self-help books, that what I was feeling was grief. What I knew about grief is that it tends to get worse before it gets better. I could be in for a long wait. My mind felt like it had been hijacked with no glimmer of clarity.

I was way too exhausted to even think about divorce. Survival was my number one priority, and to pay my share on our marital property, as well as my rental property. I have always been a firm believer in kindness and fairness, whatever the situation. Those values run deeply through my veins, and there was no way I wanted to leave my husband in a mess with the household finances now that he was living there alone.

I could keep everything going for now – I had to. I worked hard and long hours, throwing myself into my client projects. I loved my job, and I needed the money, but I also wanted to feel safe, loved and secure, and I wasn't sure I would ever feel any of those things again.

There were many wobbly days, but I always knew I had the strength and belief within me to heal from the inside out. I reminded myself I wasn't broken – I never had been. I'd just lost my way and couldn't see the beauty within myself right now.

Each day, I pushed myself hard. I went out, even when I didn't want to. I smiled when I was crying inside. I cycled and walked when all I wanted to do was curl up on the sofa and watch TV. I wrote my feelings down: the good, the bad and the ugly, ending each day by giving myself a pat on the back for something I had achieved. It could be anything, however small. I might have talked to someone new in my town, won a business contract, or even assembled a piece of IKEA furniture. Anything to do with DIY got extra self-praise! I have never been the practical kind…and that's OK!

I knew everything would work itself out because it usually does in the end. Even in my darkest moments, a deep part of me had full realisation that amid the mire and all the angst, I was alright. I always had been.

It wasn't too long before I was thriving.

I felt great. I noticed I was smiling and laughing more. I was sleeping better and had started to put on some much-needed weight. My shaky hands were steadier, and my eyes shone. I had tons of energy and looked happy and healthy.

I made lots of new friends and became familiar with my new town. I loved the ease of its great location and fast rail links into London. Slowly but surely, I had created my new normal.

My biggest realisation was that I felt at one with myself. I was at peace and comfortable in my own skin.

I had fallen in love with myself.

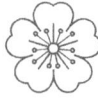

Chapter 18

Love Again

Isn't it ironic that we often miss what is right under our nose? My future partner was right there – had been for years – and I didn't see it coming.

To me, that was movie stuff. I loved the idea of falling in love again, but how often does that happen in the real world?

I had lost count of how many Christmases I had sat with a glass of wine and a Chocolate Orange, tears rolling down my cheeks, in front of my favourite romantic movies: *Sleepless in Seattle, An Affair to Remember, Falling in Love, Love Story* and *Terms of Endearment.* I loved the characters in those amazing classics, the way they would follow their truth, create their own destiny. They navigated the heady mix of physical and mental attraction. Each connection led to its passionate climax and the dream ticket we all long for: Love, respect and friendship.

Bill was my colleague and my work best friend. We had been friends since our companies had merged five years before.

We met at the launch conference in Rome. The Marriott

Hotel Reception coffee machine had been the location of our first hello.

"You must be in the other company because I don't recognise you? Would you like a coffee?" I said.

He had smiled and asked for a white coffee with two sugars.

I continued to waffle, one of my Liz traits. "My boss told me to go and mingle, meet the new folks," I said with a cheeky grin.

That comment was a tad emotive, given the fact that my company had acquired his company, taking no prisoners along the way.

"Yes, my boss said the same to me," he replied smiling, adding, "who cares less about that shit anyway? Tell me about you."

That was how our friendship started: innocent and jovial.

The connection was instant. We were both married, and we lived at opposite ends of the British Isles but had similar jobs and similar outlooks on life. We made each other laugh and both had a cheeky, dry sense of humour with barrel loads of banter, at a time when not many people in the business were laughing.

We helped each other. We had each other's backs, particularly when one of us was feeling the pressure. We spoke on the phone most days. We shared our hopes and our fears, our vulnerabilities, and sometimes we shared our lunch! It was simple, easy, and authentic.

Years passed, and it was a bombshell when my redundancy letter arrived. I had been expecting it, but it was still a shock. I wasn't too bothered about losing the job, but I had been bothered about losing contact with my best mate. That would have been a bitter pill to swallow. I soon moved on and embraced a fresh start in another business consultant role. Bill and I kept in touch by phone over the course of the following year.

Bill seemed shocked and concerned when I told him I had left my husband and moved south. I think he was worried about me and could hear I wasn't coping well. As soon as we were able to meet up and have a proper chat, we did. We found a cute little pub on the canalside where we talked for hours. I got very emotional. He was a good listener.

Bill's marriage had also broken down. We had made an emotional connection long before, and our friendship had given us a solid foundation. We were both free and ready to take our relationship to a new level. We figured there was no harm in giving it a go, but we were most definite that if it didn't work out, we had to stay friends – our friendship could not be compromised.

Our romantic partnership developed at a fast pace. We loved each other's company and were rarely apart. We both had a dry sense of humour and knew how to make each other laugh. It always felt like we were on the same side, and we had huge respect for each other.

We moved into a rental apartment together at the beginning, to be sure we had done the right thing. To our surprise, our routine was quite straightforward. There was no doubt we were compatible. The only snag was that neither of us was great at cooking, but we soon mastered that. We started with easy dishes and gave each other lots of praise, even when the meals didn't taste that good. It is amazing what you can create when you put your mind to it. Before long, we were surprising ourselves with our culinary creations.

We grew out of our tiny flat after about a year. We both missed open green space and a front door that opened onto ground level. Not to mention the challenges we'd had with underground car parking spaces. The rental had served us well though and will always hold a special place in our hearts.

I now had the strength and courage to finalise my divorce and to buy another house.

I wasn't alone. Bill would be with me every step of the way. He was my rock and best mate.

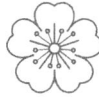

Chapter 19

A Village Less Ordinary

Stick a pin in the map, draw a ten-mile circle around it, and phone an estate agent. It was as easy as that – in theory anyway!

We knew we wanted to live in the country, but we had some caveats. We had to be within an hour of London and Heathrow for business, and within an hour of my mum in the Midlands.

Those rigid stipulations meant that we dropped our pin over the market town of Thame, Oxfordshire, a few miles from the Northern Buckinghamshire border. Feeling satisfied with our planning process, we had set off, equipped with notepad and road atlas. We were on a mission to find our dream home.

We loved Thame. It was a bustling town which felt just the right size. It had a cattle market, a quaint town hall and a wide variety of restaurants, bars and trendy boutiques. Despite – or perhaps because of – its perfection, the property prices were extortionate, and we figured we needed to extend our search across county boundaries into Northern Buckinghamshire.

We made a mental note to express interest in other towns and villages around the county periphery. We indulged in a long loop of a drive, which gave us a good feel for the area. I had the perfect property in my mind: A barn conversion on a village green, with a pub, shop and church nearby.

I was desperate for a garden. I missed having somewhere to sunbathe and barbeque in the summer and longed to have another dog. After a day exploring, we returned home tired, but upbeat. We had dropped into five estate agents to express our interest and leave our details. Now we needed the phone to start ringing.

It wasn't long before we were inundated with house brochures and phone calls. After narrowing it down to four or five possibilities, we scheduled a day to look around several properties in rural Buckinghamshire. I adore looking inside people's homes. Being naturally nosy, it was fascinating entertainment.

When we arrived at the estate agents on that frosty October morning, the agent informed us he had secured eight viewings for us, which would take up most of the day. It was very exciting. We knew we would know instantly when we found the right house, and neither of us pondered too long on our decisions.

My motto is: *when you know, you know.* Bill was exactly the same. We were about to spend a lot of money though and didn't want to make a mistake. On that note, we agreed to engage our heads, as well as our hearts, on our house-hunting mission.

House number five, out of a possible eight, was the one. I knew it as soon as we pulled up on the drive of the neat, Victorian cottage with its pretty period features, overlooking the village green onto open fields. It had a wealth of character with exposed beams and braced doors. In the cosy lounge was an open fire with a feature brick fireplace and solid oak floors. The jewel in the crown for me was the Aga in the traditional farmhouse kitchen. I had always wanted one, ever since I was a little girl. My sister and I used to warm our bottoms on Grandma's as we watched her bake. It brought back so many childhood memories.

As soon as I entered the cottage, I said, "This is it. I am home. I feel it, Bill. We have to buy this cottage."

I'd got a palpable sense of belonging which I couldn't ignore. The cottage felt as if it was pulling us in. I considered whether it might be haunted, surmising that even if there were spirits present, they meant us no harm.

It was a reassuring thought. Bill was just as taken with it as I was. We put in an offer the same day. Our heads and hearts knew it was the right decision.

Twelve weeks later, we moved into our dream home. We were so excited, yet neither of us fully appreciated that this wasn't just a new home – we had bought into a new life.

The village we had chosen would turn our lives around forever. We had both been brought up in city suburbs, where you might know your neighbours a little bit, but you don't really know anyone. We had got used to living that same reality in our home in the southeast. Our typical routine would be to go to our local pub on a Friday evening, grab a bar stool, and catch up with each other about our week. No one would listen, or butt in. No one really cared.

Here, in this village, however, things couldn't have been more different.

We went to the local pub on our first Friday evening in the village. We did our usual thing. We sat on the high bar stools and ordered our drinks. For me, a glass of chilled white wine and a packet of mini cheddars. For Bill, a pint of lager and a bag of dry-roasted peanuts. Within seconds, people started to talk to us. They even asked us to move our stools around so we looked into the pub, not into the bar. They asked us where we had moved from, what we did for a living, how long we had been together, and whether we were married. Why had we picked this village? Had we got any kids or dogs?

Their questions seemed endless and a little invasive. Were all villages like this? So nosy? Were they rude? Were they just friendly? It was perplexing. Neither of us could answer those questions. It felt like we were famous, or a novelty.

Having lived in the village for eleven years now, I know it's just how villages are, or rather, this village, anyway! We weren't anything special. The locals were just curious and wanted to know everything, and they were good people who couldn't do enough for us. Dinner invitations rolled in. That was quite a shock to the system at first, because it meant we had to reciprocate. Though we were getting better, we weren't up to dinner party cooking standards – nowhere close!

We both joined committees in the first year: Bill, the Parish Council; and me, the village fete committee, and the church cleaning rota.

My uncle thought it was hilarious. He joked that I would be making jam for the Women's Institute next! Cheeky!...

I wasn't that old, but I did want to do my bit in my new community. This was our fresh start, and I felt blessed to be living in a village crossed between the *Vicar of Dibley* and *Midsomer Murders*. As Grandma always used to say, "If you can't beat them, you might as well join them, darling." That is exactly what we did, and soon the months rolled into years. We have made fantastic friends, whom we will cherish for life. We are now blessed to have our plus one: our spoilt golden retriever, Lexi – a gorgeous country girl, through and through.

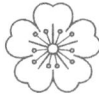

Chapter 20

Love and Loss

30th June 2016.

I couldn't have felt happier. Everything had fallen into place. I was on cloud nine. Bill, whom I loved with all my heart, had proposed on our favourite beach. I had to pinch myself as it hadn't seemed real.

We were on holiday on the Isle of Iona, a tiny Hebridean island in Northwest Scotland. He had waited until we were strolling along the familiar, deserted white sand beach on the northern tip of the island. He got down on one knee, took my hands in his, and looked straight into my eyes. As he proposed, he presented me with a diamond solitaire ring.

I was so shocked and excited. I can't remember his exact words, but I do remember the look of love and tenderness in his dark navy eyes. His expression was hopeful and ready. As if I would turn him down!

I had waited for this moment for a long time. I gleamed from ear to ear as I took in the words, my eyes filled with tears, as I threw my head back, and shouted my answer high into the grey Scottish sky.

"Yes, yes, please!" I shrieked with joy, jumping up and down and skipping into the freezing Atlantic waves, which crashed against my bare shins. I was getting married again. I had been given a second chance to get things right. I wasn't a bad person after all…

The excitement had been overwhelming. So many thoughts and questions had rushed through my head. *Who to tell? What to say? When and where would the big day be?*

Of all the days to have almost zero mobile phone signal!

Top of the list to hear our news was Mum. She could barely hear me, but even through the patchy signal, she felt my excitement and was treated to every intimate detail.

From their very first meeting, she had adored Bill, and I remember feeling her tears of love and happiness as they almost trickled through the phone. Mum and I had gotten really close after Dad had died five years before, our mutual realisation being that she had needed me as much as I had needed her over those last turbulent years.

After the blissful proposal, we were blessed with an interesting evening.

Of course, naturally, we had a romantic picture in mind. Alas, our idyllic night was not to be: our campfire was too damp, and, despite our best efforts, it was impossible to keep it alight.

We were too high on life to care and ravished a hearty fish and chip supper, washed down with some flat champagne.

There was a fierce Atlantic storm overnight, and our tent

blew down at 2 am. We were cold and wet in the howling wind and rain, so we slept fully clothed, cocooned, like Egyptian mummies, in our thermal sleeping bags. Despite the elements, we laughed like teenagers as we scrambled out of our sleeping bags to retrieve our scattered belongings, heading for the shelter of the car for the remainder of the night.

After the engagement and the storm, something inside me kept telling me to get back home and talk to Mum. I had a strong urge to see her. The journey back couldn't have been more drawn out. There was accident after accident on the M6 motorway. Mile after tedious mile of delays and speed restrictions. After a ten-hour trip, we arrived home, hot and sticky but pleased to be back in our cottage, which our village friends had decorated with welcoming balloons and banners.

It was humid that summer. Our immediate plan was to head straight up the garden to the comfortable egg chairs on our sun deck to take full advantage of the last half hour of sun. It was a delicious feeling as we sank deep into the warm, padded cushions with a cold glass of wine. I felt relaxed, with a calm sense of inner peace. I was looking forward to seeing Mum the following day to start making wedding plans. If there was one thing Mum loved, it was making plans.

As I sat there smiling, my eyes half shut, a hedgehog plodded across the middle of the lawn. It looked out of place on a sunny, mid-summer, late afternoon. It didn't seem to have a care in the world. The image prompted me to phone Mum a little earlier than I had planned to. She loved hedgehogs. As children, we always used to feed them in the garden, making sure there was a warm, comfortable box ready in the shed for when it got cold, and they were ready to hibernate.

Still wearing my holiday flip flops, I strode down the lawn into the house. It felt cool and inviting, but with a hint of muskiness, having been shut up for a week. I grabbed the landline phone and flopped down onto the slouchy sofa. Mum answered the phone on the second ring. I smiled as I heard her voice. "You're back, darling. I am so happy for you. I have told everyone. This is going to be the best wedding. Did you have a date in mind?"

"Yes," I answered, "June next year."

"That long?" she said, sounding surprised. "I hope I'm still around," she said, laughing at her flippant remark. She had always worried about getting old, but at seventy-four, she was as fit as a fiddle, had the figure of a forty-year-old, and had more energy than any of her friends.

I scolded her dark humour, going on to say I didn't want anything massive. "Just a small do for close friends and immediate family," I said.

"OK sweetheart," she said in a happy tone.

I asked her what she had planned for her evening. The response was silence... a crackly line, heavy breathing... gasping. Then nothing.

"Mum, Mum!" I shouted, my voice getting louder and more urgent.

Still nothing, more crackles, then silence. I felt sick. I had palpitations.

I was sweating profusely.

I knew.

Every fibre of my being resisted the idea, but I knew she had just died.

I knew I was right…

Bill heard my shouts and rushed into the room, a concerned look on his face.

"What's up?" he asked. "I can hear you at the top of the garden."

I looked at him with horror. My eyes were wide, like black saucers.

My bottom lip quivered, and my voice trembled.

I answered in a whisper. "It's Mum…"

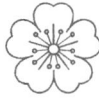

Chapter 21

Grief

After Mum's death, I was heartbroken, confused and lost. Everything I had taken for granted was gone.

It was harder because Mum and I had become so much closer since Dad's death. We had both realised how precious life is and how precarious it can be.

We had never expected our strong, healthy Dad to become ill. He only lived for one year after his cancer diagnosis. That devastating reality made Mum, Jane and I closer than we had ever been.

Just after Dad died, we kept a close eye on Mum and, slowly but surely, we watched her find her wings. To our surprise, she wanted to do things she would never have dreamed of doing on her own when Dad was alive. She travelled across the world, exploring America and India. She treated herself to a new car, a metallic cream Mini, which she named Daisy.

She project-managed a garage conversion and re-designed the garden.

It had been inspiring to watch her confidence grow. She

always maintained she was "carrying on," as opposed to "moving on." Mum was our very own Wonder Woman, and we adored her for it. She was glowing from the inside out.

For five years, we watched Mum with pride as she created her new life. Just when we thought she had found peace, with an appreciation of her own inner strength and beauty, she suffered a catastrophic brain haemorrhage: in layman's terms, a bleed to the brain. She never regained consciousness. She died happy, in her favourite leather armchair, on that warm July afternoon, phone in hand, talking to me.

The first few weeks after her death remain a bit of a blur. I remember the utter shock and emptiness. Endless phone calls. Copious amounts of paperwork and organising. Permanent exhaustion. I waited for the tears, but they never came.

I kept myself busy during the day, but the nights seemed like endless blackness. I was haunted by her image and that last phone call, waking night after night, breathless, coated in a cold sweat. I would pace around the bedroom like a trapped animal. My question was always, *Why? Why now? Was I being punished by a higher power for leaving my previous life and starting afresh?* I had no answers, but my overactive mind tortured me.

By the end of August, I felt numb and couldn't make sense of anything. Mum was in my head, my heart, my dreams, my daily consciousness. She was everywhere. She was dead, and I couldn't accept it.

Bill was amazing. With his unconditional love and natural ability to keep me calm in a crisis, he helped me face my demons. He listened to my endless rants, accepted the angry outbursts when they appeared, with gentle kindness and a soothing hug. We both knew I was experiencing the usual stages of grief, but when you are in the middle of it, it is not as easy as reading about it in a book.

I got there in the end. I had no choice. Life goes on, whether we are ready for it or not. I had proved that to myself time and time again. I was more resilient than I thought.

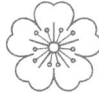

Chapter 22

A Change of Scene

By the end of September, we needed a change of scene.

We took off for a fortnight. We visited Bill's brother in Mexico City for a few days and then, from there, headed over to Cabo San Lucas on the Baja California Peninsula in northwestern Mexico for some beach time. It was just what we needed.

There is a certain 'edginess' to Mexico, which is great for taking your mind off things, and wandering around the sprawling streets of Mexico City was a perfect distraction. Given the fact that Mexico City has a reputation for crime, our main priority was to stay safe. For the first time in three months, I wasn't thinking about Mum. It was a start!

We survived Mexico City with ease, probably because Ian was a great guide and a long-term local. We arrived in Cabo five days later feeling relaxed, fresh and hopeful. I was determined to focus on the present and make the most of the tropical paradise we had landed in.

Even though we were supposed to relax that week, I am

naturally nomadic. I soon had the maps and guidebooks spread out across the kitchen table in our beach villa, searching for idyllic places to visit. By the end of our first day, I had organised a rental Jeep and had a road trip planned for the following day. The road trip would reward us with the best bits of the Cabo Peninsula. Stunning white sand beaches, tropical forests, mountains and dramatic waterfalls awaited us. We couldn't wait!

The day started off well. The Jeep was a cute, bright red with an open top. We found our first stop, bang on schedule: Balandra Beach, a breathtaking white sand beach set in a crescent-shaped bay on the Sea of Cortez, near the busy fishing port of La Paz. The water was a crystal shade of jade, shallow and warm, and the shoreline was deserted apart from a few locals. No tourists. No Brits. What a dream! It was paradise.

We only stayed there an hour because we wanted to see more and complete our full schedule. I wanted to pack as much into the day as I could in case I never returned. We carried on with our circular loop, which took us inland, down dusty single tracks, through dense forests, into the mountains where we discovered quaint villages steeped with Mexican culture. We were well off the beaten track.

In the guidebook, I could see a famous waterfall, high in the mountains. It was a gem by all accounts, and a popular stop for the more adventurous tourists. Bill had his doubts, saying he thought it looked a little remote, and the map wasn't the clearest to follow. I was as determined as ever, pointing out that we could stop and ask for directions if we needed to.

An hour later, we entered a village with a delightful square, boasting an impressive circular fountain at its centre. I hate asking for help when on an adventure, but sometimes, needs must! We went into the village shop, both conscious of our non-existent Spanish, where we were eyed up and down by a handful of bored-looking locals who congregated in the ornate wooden doorway. We showed them our map and guidebook, and they nodded. They appeared animated and happy to help us, pointing in the direction of the steep hill which led off the village square beyond. As their English was almost non-existent, they raised two hands to let us know it would take about ten minutes to get to the waterfall by car.

Something was off. I wasn't convinced it was safe. My gut was telling me to get out of there fast. But I was too proud to abandon my mission.

We followed the road, as instructed. After about fifteen minutes, we came to a junction where we chose to go straight on and not follow the road round the bend to the right. The road turned into a rocky nightmare with boulders and craters on each side of the track. Thank goodness we had a Jeep because it was almost impassable. Not wanting to get stuck, we managed, with some effort, to turn the Jeep around, heading back towards the main road.

When we got back to the junction, we met a car that had followed us out of the village. The driver was signalling for us to follow him. This definitely didn't feel right. We both sensed trouble and we were acutely aware that we looked like tourists. It was blatantly obvious: my designer sunglasses, broadbrimmed sun hat, white shorts, strappy sun top, flip flops and Cabo beach bag, kind of gave it away!

I hadn't got as much jewellery on as I usually wear, but the diamond in my engagement ring stood out like a sore thumb on my tanned left hand, as did Bill's expensive watch on his exposed wrist.

We felt vulnerable and scared. My gut was telling me, loud and clear, that we were being led into a trap. We ignored his signal, waved politely, like most well-behaved British tourists do, and then sped past him in the opposite direction. It was like a scene out of the Dukes of Hazzard, dust flying high into the air behind us.

What might have happened will remain a mystery, but something was not right. I had gone as far as taking my engagement ring off and hiding it down my knickers, only retrieving it when we were back on a built-up main road! Not that it would have made any difference if we had been attacked. It is funny what we do when we feel under threat and what we think we value most. I know my engagement ring would have been the last thing on my mind if I had been assaulted!

Back in the hotel bar, with our drama behind us, we laughed, celebrating our safe return with a tequila shot each. The more I laughed, the more I couldn't stop laughing out of sheer relief. Then, from nowhere, came the tears. They poured down my flushed cheeks, plopping like salty raindrops into my tequila.

I had waited so long for those tears.

I wanted my Mum.

She was gone.

Part Two

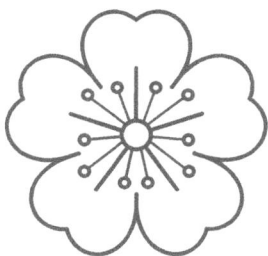

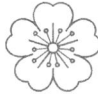

Chapter 23

The Cancer

September 2022.

I couldn't put my finger on it, but I didn't feel quite right.

I wasn't feeling light on my feet and had an intermittent dull ache in my lower right side, which would occasionally cramp in spasms, making me wince. I felt like someone was stapling me from the inside.

Not being one to give in to anything without a fight, I had put on a brave face as I planned our annual trip to California. When we boarded the plane, on a cool autumn morning, I didn't feel my usual holiday excitement, however. Something was wrong. I sensed it, and I dreaded it.

We had a good fortnight, despite my pain. The first five days were spent in Lake Tahoe, which had been on our to-do list for years, our previous trips having been cancelled several times throughout the pandemic.

As we adapted to Pacific time, we lay in bed in the early hours of the morning and watched the Queen's funeral on the huge American television. It occurred to me what a full and long life our Queen had had. Her loyal service and duty were her core defining legacy. I watched the service in awe, not quite able to shrug off the feeling that I was ill. My intuition told me to seek medical advice as soon as I got home.

We returned to the UK on October 2nd, and the next day, my mission to understand what was wrong with me began.

October 3rd marked the first day of what would become seven months of frustration and uncertainty. Between October 2022 and the end of April 2023, I had four telephone and three face-to-face consultations with my family doctor.

Each discussion ended with the usual, "I don't think you have anything to worry about, Liz, this looks like nothing more serious than a flare-up of irritable bowel syndrome (IBS). It's very common and easy to manage with medication. You need to relax about it. You seem very anxious."

I spent a lot of money on anti-spasmodic and laxative medications, to no avail.

By May 2023, I couldn't stand it any longer. I made the decision to self-refer to a private consultant gastroenterologist. It felt good to take action, but I suspected my GP thought I was a hypochondriac.

I was anxious on the day of the clinic appointment, but felt reassured when the consultant took my symptoms seriously. She was professional and kind, and recommended two scoping procedures.

The colonoscopy and gastroscopy weren't as bad as I expected them to be. I was sedated for each. Much to my relief, each of these tests, and all my blood tests, were normal. A confusing outcome, as it didn't answer why I felt so much pain. Maybe my family doctor had been right after all?

Reassured by that conclusion, I relaxed. I was going to be OK. The thought was short-lived though, as the consultant recommended I get a CT scan of my abdomen and pelvis: "Just to be safe. To check for lumps and bumps. I don't expect to see anything," she said, smiling at me, with a gentle squeeze of my shoulder.

A week later, I returned for my results. I felt good as we had just returned from a long weekend in Portugal, and I was pleased to tell her I was feeling much better. Perhaps everything had been in my head after all?

Once again, I sat before this personable consultant, who welcomed me with a smile and a strong handshake.

"I am feeling great," I said, before she had a chance to say anything.

"That's good to hear, Liz. We have your CT scan result. You have a five-centimetre cyst on your right ovary. That is a big cyst for your small frame. We should get a gynaecologist to see you. They will likely want to remove it via keyhole surgery. Cysts are very common. Don't worry, it's likely to be nothing."

"Oh," I said, rather taken aback. "Is that why I have been getting pain on my right side? Would a cyst create that amount of pain?"

"Yes," she said, "very likely, but let's get you seen as soon as possible by the gynae team. Leave it with me to organise."

I wouldn't say I was devastated by the news because ovarian

cysts are common, and often harmless, but I had mixed feelings.

The first was relief: Thank goodness they had found the root cause of my pain. The second feeling was more of a fear of the unknown. What if the cyst was sinister? At fifty-four, I was post-menopausal, and cysts are more common in women who haven't been through menopause. I had sold a chemotherapy agent for ovarian cancer when I worked in the pharmaceutical industry, and wondered if a little knowledge might well be a dangerous thing. I tried to stay off Google, but like anything I know I shouldn't do, it was hard to resist the temptation. I found myself drawn into a myriad of internet data.

It was late June when the nightmare started in earnest.

A radiologist performed a pelvic ultrasound scan. There was a look of horror on her face as she described my ovarian mass as, "complex, suspicious and requiring an urgent gynae-cological oncology opinion." I spiralled into a blind panic while I underwent a week of tests, including a second CT scan, an MRI scan, and a panel of tumour marker blood tests.

Results day was scheduled for July 17th.

I was hysterical with panic. My mood would flip in an instant. One moment, I would be philosophical and practical about matters; the next, I would feel overwhelmed and be in floods of tears.

Poor Bill didn't know what to say for the best, bless him. He refused to believe I had cancer until he was told. His ethos was that we would deal with it together if, and when, we needed to. Nights dragged with insomnia. My mind raced with every possible scenario. It was hell waiting for the results to come back. I couldn't help but fear the worst.

Results day came. The wait in the outpatient lounge seemed endless. My mouth was dry. I couldn't find any words to make conversation with Bill. Eventually, we were called into the consulting room.

I knew it was bad news before my consultant opened his mouth. He told me I had cancer. I heard the words, but they didn't feel real. I felt like I was having an out-of-body experience. His words sounded like echoes in a bottomless cave. He told me a multi-disciplinary team of radiologists, surgeons and oncologists had looked at my scans, and the consensus was that I had extensive stage three ovarian cancer. I would require an urgent hysterectomy with cytoreductive surgery to remove the tumour, followed by chemotherapy after the operation. Cytoreductive surgery is a technique where all diseased body tissue is removed.

The only good news was that the cancer appeared to be low-grade. That meant the cancer cells had grown very slowly over a long period of time. As devastating as this news was to absorb, it still didn't feel like it was happening.

I sat quietly, looking at him, listening to every word.

When he finished talking, I said, "I understand. I take it you can cure me. I am not ready to die. I will do whatever is needed."

With equal calmness, he answered, "We can treat this Liz. The operation is big, and we may find more spread when we look inside your abdomen. Chemotherapy doesn't tend to work well with low-grade cancers. Your best option is surgery, but there are no guarantees. I am sorry."

His words were devastating. I needed some hope. He was still looking at my blood tumour markers.

"Are all my blood tests abnormal?" I asked, my voice croaky.

"Your CEA tumour marker is very high, which would indicate that your bowel might be affected." After a pause, he went on to say he wasn't one hundred per cent convinced the cancer was of ovarian origin, despite the team's conclusions. He had a feeling something else might be at play in my abdominal region.

"You mean I might have bowel cancer as well?" I stammered in disbelief.

"I am not sure. The raised tumour marker could be a red herring," he said, as he continued to study my results, shaking his head. With that question in mind, he told me to play it safe; he would do an exploratory laparoscopy first, before the big operation. This would give him a thorough look inside my abdomen and pelvis with a camera, before he removed anything.

He wanted to anaesthetise me for the eight-hour full surgery, even though he wasn't convinced by the diagnosis. The final decision on how to proceed would be made during the laparoscopy, while I was asleep on the operating table.

I arrived home that evening with a heavy heart. I had three weeks to wait until the operation. More sheep to count at 3 am. More episodes of *Frasier* to stare at blankly. More weight I'd lose, as I was struggling to eat even the tiniest of meals. And the most depressing thought of all: more paperwork to sort through, as I couldn't shake the thought that I wouldn't survive the operation.

After what seemed an eternity, the morning of August 10th arrived. I felt nervous as I sat in my dressing gown on the edge of the hospital bed. I had scrubbed my face clean and removed my earrings, but couldn't bring myself to remove my wedding ring. I felt closer to Bill with it on. I shared my feelings with the kind nurse, and she smiled as she lifted my left hand and gently wrapped surgical tape across the ring on my frail third finger. Physically, I was ready to go into theatre. Psychologically, I was not ready to deal with what they might find. I felt powerless, in disbelief that it had come to this.

I didn't know whether I was going in for an eight-hour operation or a one-hour procedure. I didn't know whether I would wake up. If I didn't wake, I wondered whether I would go to heaven or hell. What I did know is that I wanted to live.

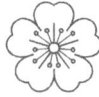

Chapter 24

What the F*** is Pseudomyxoma Peritonei?

"Hi Liz, wake up, sweetheart. You are in recovery; you have had your operation."

I came to, feeling groggy, my throat sore, and my head spinning. The ceiling light in the recovery room was harsh. The bright rays stung my heavy eyes.

"What time is it?" I said to the nurse.

"It is 10.30 am Liz. We will take you back to your room in about fifteen minutes."

"How can it only be 10.30 am?" I said, a lump in the back of my throat.

"I was supposed to be under for eight hours. I don't understand. Have they not done the surgery?"

My voice had become high-pitched and hysterical. I couldn't push away the feeling of dread. I had gone into the operating theatre at 9 am, an hour and a half earlier.

"Try to relax Liz," the nurse said in a soft voice.

"Your surgeon will come and talk to you when you are back in your room."

How the hell could I relax? I concluded that they had inserted the camera into my abdomen and found extensive, inoperable cancer. There must be no hope! My mind was racing as I attempted to predict my fate, even though I was still heavily sedated. My limbs felt like lead weights, and my head was throbbing. My adrenaline wanted to flow, but it felt like it was being blocked by the anaesthetic. It reminded me of being in a nightmare, trying to run up a staircase covered in glue, but instead of climbing, I was sinking into each sticky stair.

No surprise, really. I had been anaesthetised on the assumption it would be an eight-hour surgery.

Fifteen minutes later, I was back in my room. My body felt rigid as I lay on my back, my eyes fixed on a blemish on the pale green ceiling. Bill had been telephoned and was on his way. What on earth could I tell him? I knew nothing, but in my head, the writing was on the wall. I was near death. They couldn't help me.

I felt sick. He would be devastated. My eyes filled with tears as I thought about his kind, loving face and the conversation that lay ahead. Bill loved me. He would miss me when I was gone. He had been optimistic and supportive, willing me to be brave, reassuring me they would cut out all the cancer, and I would look and feel as good as new. What did he know?!

I didn't hear the surgeon when he entered the room. I was lost in my thoughts and had a strange sensation that I was floating above my body. The dissociative effect of the ketamine was doing its job; just one of the potent ingredients in my anaesthetic cocktail.

"Liz," he said, his tone soft and gentle. I jumped when I heard his voice, turning my head towards him. My watery green eyes studied his soft brown eyes. I searched for answers, looked for hope. "What happened?" I said.

"We got a big surprise Liz, when we looked inside your abdomen. You don't have ovarian cancer. Your ovaries are healthy. You do have cancer, but it is coming from your appendix. You have a disease called Pseudomyxoma Peritonei (PMP), it's a form of appendix cancer. Your appendix has ruptured and spread mucin, which is a jellylike substance, around your whole abdomen. That is what has been causing your pain. The jelly fluid has been pressing on your internal abdominal organs, including your bowel and your right ovary. This is a very rare type of cancer, Liz. One in a million cases, and it is hard to diagnose. It often doesn't show up on scans or in blood samples. It is treatable, but we can't operate here. You will have to go to Basingstoke Hospital. It is a world-class centre that specialises in peritoneal cancers. They will look after you. This is a treatable disease and, potentially, the operation is curative. Trust me, this might be a shock, but this disease has a more positive prognosis than ovarian cancer. I will ask the nurse to write the information down for you. I have arranged for the lead surgeon from Basingstoke to phone you tomorrow afternoon to arrange a date for your surgery. You can leave here tomorrow morning. Do you understand what I have told you? I will explain everything to Bill when he arrives."

I struggled to take in all the information, but even in my

drugged state, I had a question. "OK, thanks for explaining everything. I need some time to take this in. How long do you think I have had this for?"

His reply still astonishes me to this day. "You have probably had it for about ten years, Liz. It is a very slow-growing cancer. Often, there are no symptoms. You are young and fit, so you should get through this and go on to make a full recovery."

"Ten years!" I gasped. *How the hell did I not know there had been something growing inside my tummy for ten years?*

With that, he was gone; his work was done.

I still had a hell of a journey ahead of me.

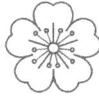

Chapter 25

The Mother of All Surgeries

I returned home the next morning.

Oddly, I felt elated. As strange as it might sound, I felt I had been given a chance. After months of uncertainty, there was a diagnosis. I had clarity. I reasoned that, yes, this was a rare disease, and yes, it was a type of appendix cancer, but somehow, I felt saved. The cancer could be removed. I was going to a specialist centre to get the gold standard of care. It was that simple.

The operation was called cyto-reductive surgery with hyperthermic intraperitoneal chemotherapy (CRS+HIPEC). It was also known, in the clinical world, as the Mother of All Surgeries (MOAS) and would take around nine hours. After the initial removal of the abdominal organs affected by the PMP, my abdomen would then be flushed with the HIPEC, which is a heated form of chemotherapy that kills any remaining cancer cells that might be lurking, undetectable to the human eye.

I would then be kept in an induced coma in the Intensive Care Unit for around twenty-four hours following the operation, and remain in hospital for two to three weeks. What was there to worry about?!

I had no idea how huge the operation would be, and the impact it would have on me physically and psychologically. My surgeon had warned me that full recovery would take around two years. I was somewhat detached from the full reality. My mind was protecting me from the full, gruesome details of the situation. To be honest, though, I think that's how I got through it. I chose to minimise it. I didn't want sympathy or attention, and made the choice to limit those who knew to my sister, best friend, employer, ex-husband, and a couple of close friends in our village. I stuck to the facts and kept the details top line. I had no control over the cancer, but I could control the story I shared, and I exercised that privilege. My body, my rules, my life.

On the morning of the operation, despite my nerves, I resigned myself to the fact that I was in their hands; this tiny, vulnerable, sick version of me. I fell into unconsciousness after hearing the anaesthetist's words, "Just another day in the office for me…"

It was obvious that his comment was supposed to reassure me. It didn't!

That was my last thought as I felt myself fall, fall, fall, away into nothingness.

This time around, I got the operation I was promised. I woke up twenty-four hours later, minus my appendix, spleen, ovaries, uterus, gall bladder and a small section of my large bowel. As drastic as that sounds, I can still live a healthy life without any of these organs.

I was told the operation had taken just under nine hours. It had been successful, and all the disease had been removed.

The heated chemotherapy had been flushed through my abdomen while I was under anaesthetic. I wouldn't know whether I needed to have any additional (traditional) systemic chemotherapy until the histology results were back from the lab.

I had a long, neat, stapled cut that started under my chest and ran down to my pubic bone. I was fed through an intravenous drip for ten days. I had an annoying naso-gastric tube up my nose, which created constant irritation in the back of my throat. There were four drains protruding from my chest and abdomen. I was in a bad way, but the cancer was gone, and that was all I cared about. I was alive and, much to my relief, I had escaped the need for a stoma.

The two weeks that followed were pure hell – a nightmare. The pain was unbearable. I was exhausted. Any movement, even blinking, felt like an effort. On my third day in ICU, my haemoglobin levels dropped, and I needed an urgent blood transfusion. My blood pressure remained "dangerously higher than normal."

I would wake up, screaming in agony, my nightdress damp with sweat, twisted around my tiny, depleted body. The nausea and sickness were a constant; and the nights, endless and black. All night, I could see the flickering patterns of the red and green lights on the complex display monitors in the windowless ICU room. I couldn't get comfortable in any position.

Sitting up and walking were only possible with assistance. Each morning, the physiotherapists would arrive smiling at 10 am, lift me from my bed to the chair, and then, with the help of a frame, make me practice walking down the corridor. They pushed me hard. Every excruciating step was a personal triumph. I tried to be brave and get on with it. My pride and resilience were still intact, but there were moments when I felt it would be easier to die.

On good days, I would dream about my bucket list. I would make travel plans in my head, imagine I was spinning my globe, fantasising about every possibility. I would acknowledge what I had already achieved, giving myself a pat on the back for the places I had been to in my life. I appreciated how blessed I had been to find love and inner peace.

On the bad days, I saw blackness: No future. No hope. A life of pain and uncertainty.

My life had been turned upside down, my body ripped apart.

There were no in-between days. It was either black or white.

Bill held my hand almost twenty-four seven throughout my whole stay in ICU.

Eventually, my discharge day came, along with the histology results from the lab.

"Thank fuck for that," I shouted when the surgeon shared my results, a broad beam lighting up his kind face.

"It's low-grade, Liz. We thought it was, but it is great to get it confirmed by the lab. That means no more chemotherapy

– you are cured. We got all the cancer. You are going to be OK. You can go home."

Bless him, he seemed so happy to share the news. I thought about how tough it must be for doctors to share results. It must be rewarding for them, too, when things work out well. "Thank you, thank you, so, so much, for everything." I blurted through tears.

Then off he went, after telling me that he would see me in the outpatients' clinic in six weeks' time.

I was elated. I was done.

In silence, I allowed Bill to lift me into the wheelchair that had been placed at the side of my bed, in preparation for our departure.

We were on our way home.

Back to the cottage.

A long recovery lay ahead.

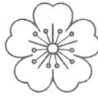

Chapter 26

Soup, Cake and Morphine

If I could have got away with telling no one about my cancer, it would have suited me down to the ground. It is not that I didn't appreciate the love and support from my friends and family – I did. But I felt like it was a weakness to be ill. The more I was forced to talk about it, the worse it made me feel.

For the first two weeks after my discharge, I couldn't face having any visitors. I was in constant pain and needed support with basic hygiene and going to the toilet. Eating was a lottery: sometimes, food would stay down; and other times, it would come straight back up again. I was told the constant nausea and sickness were a side effect of the HIPEC chemotherapy.

I was pretty much bed-bound, getting up for about an hour each day to exercise my legs. They looked like they were wasting away, speckled with bluish green bruises from the daily blood thinning jab I had to inject into my thighs. My bottom had almost disappeared, too.

For years, I had wished for a smaller bottom. Mine had always been quite curvy and round, but when it disappeared altogether, I found myself wanting it back. I had always been petite and curvy. Now, even my extra small knickers were slipping down. My backside was so flat you could have fried a pancake on it. With so much lost muscle tone, every part of my body was smaller. Even the size six jeans Bill had ordered for me looked baggy.

One afternoon, Bill found me in a crumpled heap on the bedroom floor, surrounded by piles of clothes, sobbing hard because nothing fitted me anymore. He sat down and, without a word, held me close. I knew he was holding back his own tears as he listened to my loud sobs.

I lived from day to day, in elasticated tracksuit bottoms with extra-large T-shirts to disguise the fact I couldn't wear a bra because it was too painful around my upper abdominal area. Visitors were a definite no-no: No bra, no visitors!

The first two months were a challenging time. My daily walk up and down the garden would exhaust me. Only morphine would take away the searing abdominal and back pain, but the morphine also had side effects. It made the sickness worse, so it wasn't ideal. I soon abandoned it altogether, opting for paracetamol every four hours. Sitting on the sofa was painful. I couldn't get comfortable in any position. Even when I lay flat, I could feel layer upon layer of internal stitching stretching.

Agony! Nothing could have prepared me for the pain I suffered. I had been cut in half and gutted like a fish!

After a month, my weight became dangerously low. My family doctor referred me to a dietitian. The dietitian told me to eat as much protein, fat and sugar as possible. Cheese, chicken, peanut butter, cake, biscuits, white wine and full-fat milkshakes all made the grade on the goodies list. I had fifteen kilos to gain to get back to my original weight and usual size ten to twelve dress size.

That is when the kindness of our village friends really kicked in. Endless homemade soups in every flavour arrived in the poshest of village Tupperware. Homemade cakes in abundance, too. There was so much soup and cake that we had to freeze most of it. My favourites were the ginger and parsnip soup and the peanut butter chocolate squares, yum! Thank you, Naomi and Elly – you are both dear friends and great feeders!

The weight gain was slow at first. About a kilo a month, but the diet did work, and by early December, I was feeling stronger and more like myself again. We even had the odd night out. I wasn't out of the woods, though, and a return to normality seemed a long way off.

Christmas 2023 arrived early in our cottage.

I had the nagging feeling that my cancer would come back, and wondered if this might be my last Christmas. I couldn't shake off the feeling. It was a constant stone around my neck.

We both decided that distractions were important. The tree went up on November 25th, and the presents were bought and wrapped by December 1st. I went online and ordered twelve sparkly outfits, one for each day of the twelve days of Christmas.

"Might as well go out with a blast, if this is my last one," I said to Bill, who rolled his eyes, not wanting to be drawn into my irrational thinking.

"Whatever makes you happy, Baby," he said, playing it safe!

It was a magical Christmas, perfect in every way. Ross, Bill's son, came to stay with us, and the three of us, along with Lexi, our dog, made the most of every precious family moment.

Early in the New Year, I felt ready to experiment with a phased return to work. I started with two hours a day, five days a week, from home. It was tough at first. The fatigue was disabling, and there were times when I wondered whether my energy levels would ever return to the way they were. I had a clear and focused mind as I worked on my client projects, yet my body felt rigid and sore. My legs and back ached after walking the smallest of distances.

Sitting upright in my office chair or at the dinner table was challenging. I had to strengthen my core. The removal of my abdominal organs had put a strain on my back and my abdominal nerves and muscles. Every twinge in my tummy, however small, triggered a negative thought that I was getting sick again. I couldn't help the feeling of dread when I looked ahead on the calendar. August would mark my one-year anniversary, and my first twelve-month scan.

I decided to make a bucket list, or my 'Just in Case' list, as I preferred to call it.

"Things I must do before I die. I mean, I know I won't die. I'm better now. I'm doing great. But you never know. Just in case. Best to have it. No regrets and all that…" I would babble away to friends.

I was attempting to convince myself more than anyone else!

I couldn't shake the thought: *I am a dead woman walking.*

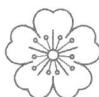

Chapter 27

Just in Case...

At first my 'Just in Case' list was short and simple. It included a handful of my favourite places in the world: California, the English Lakes and the Western Scottish Isles.

Then, I listed a couple of places I hadn't visited before: the Italian Amalfi coast, Vienna, Singapore, Australia and Western Canada. Australia was highlighted in yellow and written in capitals. I'd promised Mum I would visit sometime in my lifetime. She and Dad had adored the rich diversity of the Australian landscape and the exotic wildlife.

After completing Dad's lecture tours, they had travelled the full length of both east and west coasts. Mum made me promise I would go to Brisbane and cuddle a koala bear at the Australian zoo. I loved koala bears. The idea had always seemed so far away, and over the years, Australia had become a pipedream.

As the months passed and I got stronger, my 'Just in Case' list started to grow legs – enormous legs! It expanded across all seven continents, including a selection of European city breaks and experiences too.

I wasn't deterred. My innate, nomadic spirit and the uncertainty of my future fuelled me, full steam ahead. To Bill's credit, even though I was spending money at a frightening pace, he watched me take control of my life again, without a word of caution. He would smile, his dark blue eyes full of pride and love, as I pored over maps, spinning the globe to my heart's content.

I was back. For how long, I didn't know, but I was back for now, and I was loving it!

In the space of six months, between February and August 2024, we visited Chicago, southern Thailand, the Suffolk coast, the Isle of Arran, the Amalfi coast, the Lake District and the North Yorkshire Dales.

We got seats on Centre Court at Wimbledon – another first! It was indulgent, but we were making up for lost time. We were high on life, appreciating every moment together.

In late June, as I lay on my pool lounger, soaking up the Sorrento heat, I marvelled at the beauty of the Amalfi coast. The more I thought about it, the more curious I became as to why I hadn't visited before.

Feeling guilty and a little emotional, I picked up my phone, clicked on the Notes app and started to write.

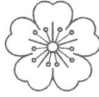

The Wait

Vertical dwellings nestle deep in cavernous limestone cliffs.
Whirls and swirls dance in flirtation on vivid turquoise water.
Gigantic lemons on the roadside.
Juicy oranges hang low and ripe, ready to make fountains of
*   Aperol Spritz.*
A slice of romantic perfection in a fast-paced, unpredictable world.
I'm captivated.
Why did I wait so long to visit the Amalfi Coast
on my European doorstep, a hop away?
I thought I had time.
To think,
I might have missed it!

Under the welcome shade of my wide-brimmed sunhat, I was conscious of how easily the words flowed from my heart. The writing felt like it was part of my natural healing process. My surroundings were exquisite, but the real beauty was coming from deep within me as my finger tapped on each letter.

As I sipped on my Aperol Spritz, there was only one dampener.

The one-year scan was six weeks away.

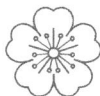

Chapter 28

Hope

August used to be my favourite month – my birthday month.

My special day always falls on or near the bank holiday weekend.

August is usually a warm month. It's a time for barbeques, weekend trips to the seaside and garden parties. While August is hot, there is often the hint of an early morning autumnal chill, a welcome addition after a long, hot summer.

August 2024 was different. It marked a year since my surgery, which meant my one-year scan was due. I started looking out for the hospital letter as soon as we returned from Italy in late June. Each morning, I listened for the post, running into our hall as soon as I heard the rattle of the letter box. I waited, but no letter arrived. Instead, on July 2nd, an email appeared.

It was a short, factual note. I read it ten times.

Dear Elizabeth,
Your CT scan and blood tests are due in August. Please

*arrive at the Radiology Department for your scan at 9 am
on August 15th. Your check-up will be in the Outpatients'
Department at 2 pm on the same day.*

I felt sick, and my hands shook as I took in the words. I
had been expecting it. I would need a yearly scan for the rest
of my life, but seeing the words in black and white made me
breathless with fear.

During the six weeks that followed, we tried to keep ourselves busy, packing our social calendar to the brim. I planned
a dinner party for eight, to be held the week before the scan to
help take my mind off things. Given that I don't have much
confidence in the kitchen, I figured that worrying about a
menu might replace the worry of the scan. The reality was
double worry! *What if the menu went wrong and my guests hated
my food? What if my cancer had come back and I faced another
operation?* Or worse: *What if the disease was terminal? What
if... What if...?!*

I was a woman possessed. I hypothesised every possibility.

The day of the appointment finally arrived. It had been
a long wait. We got up early. It was an hour and a half-long
drive. I was tired. Sleep had been a challenge, with regular
clock checks, and lots of restless tossing and turning. We didn't
speak much during the journey. I was lost in my thoughts. I
stared out of the window but saw nothing.

As we pulled into the hospital car park, my breathing had
become shallow. My palms were sweaty, and my mouth was
dry. My immediate instinct was to jump into the driver's seat,
turn the car around and get out of there fast. I wanted to be

home, snuggled up on the sofa with Lexi and a cup of tea. The memories of my long stay in ICU still haunted me. Though I said nothing, Bill reached over to squeeze my hand. We were early, so he suggested we sit in the car for a while and listen to the radio.

"No," I replied, "let's go in and do it. I'm ready," I said in a blunt tone.

I wasn't ready. As we walked into the building, I was shaking from head to toe. My wedged sandals weren't high, but I was wobbling in them, my feet clumsy. I announced my arrival at the radiology unit reception. I struggled to get my name out clearly. I was having a CT scan with contrast of my pelvis and abdomen. This meant that one hour before, I needed to have a special drink which would help highlight my intestines while being scanned. Drinking the disgusting, bitter liquid gave me something to focus on while Bill chatted away about random stuff. It was his attempt to keep my mind occupied. His easy chat was designed to keep him calm too.

After an hour, the plastic jug was empty, and I sat waiting for my name to be called, eyes transfixed on the green swing doors. There wasn't a delay, which I was grateful for. I wanted to get the scan done and get out of there, even though I had to return after lunch to see the consultant and get my results.

The radiographer was kind and calm. He helped me get my body into the correct position on the CT scanner's long flat table bed. He commented on my suntan and asked about my holidays, as he inserted an intravenous line, containing a contrast dye, into a vein in my right arm. This dye, along with the barium drink, was designed to improve visibility in my abdominal cavity. Better visibility would mean more reliable images. Frightening, but reassuring.

The scan took about fifteen minutes. As soon as he removed the line from my arm, I jumped off the bed, grabbed my shoes and handbag, and was out of there, striding at pace towards the car where I had asked Bill to meet me. I couldn't face going back into the waiting room. We had a three-and-a-half-hour wait until the consultant appointment. Every minute would feel like an eternity.

It was a warm day. The pub seemed the obvious choice to fill time. It was a five-minute drive from the hospital, and there were plenty of seats outside which overlooked a pretty stream, home to a cute family of ducks.

I wasn't hungry, but I had to eat something as I'd starved in preparation for the scan. I sat down at the nearest bench to the stream and asked Bill to order me a cheese sandwich and a glass of water. Two minutes later, he arrived back at the table with a pint of beer and a large glass of dry rosé wine. Before I could object, he said, "Liz, you need to drink this, it will take the edge off. We can't change anything now. Whatever happens, let's have a nice lunch. I've ordered you some chips too, to go with your sandwich."

He was spot on! The wine tasted good, so I had a second one, and the time passed quickly.

When we got back to the hospital, I was calmer, and the shakes had gone. I had resigned myself to *what would be, would be*. It was out of my control. I was strong, and I would accept whatever I was told.

We waited ten minutes in the outpatients' lounge, but

that was long enough. Long enough to study the faces of the staff as they went about their work. Not one of them held eye contact with us. *Was that a bad thing? Were they hiding something? What did they know?*

I didn't have long to ponder. As soon as I saw my surgeon's face, I knew I was OK. His smile was beaming. "You look great Liz, come in and have a seat."

I might be wrong, but anyone smiling like that, and telling me I looked great would surely not drop the 'C' bomb!

My theory was correct.

"Your scan is completely clear Liz. There is no evidence of disease, and your blood tests haven't shown anything either. This is great news; I don't think you will have any more problems. We will keep a good eye on you and see you again next year."

I had to ask him to repeat the words. "So, I am all clear, no cancer, at all, anywhere?" I said. I felt the relief lift from my tense body.

"Yes, Liz, completely clear, I don't think the PMP will give you any more bother."

Hearing him repeat those words was the best thing in the world. As soon as he finished speaking, I burst into tears and jumped out of my seat to give him a big hug. I didn't leave it at one hug either – there were three hugs and one kiss, to be precise!

I was exhilarated on the journey home. I let out a loud squeal of delight as we pulled out of the hospital car park. When we were about ten miles from home, I suggested we head straight to the pub and celebrate with some champagne.

I felt like the happiest and luckiest girl in the world as I sipped those delicious bubbles.

My elation lasted about a month before my emotions normalised again.

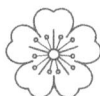

Chapter 29

Full Circle

My birthday celebrations at the end of August were extra special. There was a day trip to a health spa, a garden party with our village friends, and a romantic lunch at a posh country restaurant with Bill. I was glowing with happiness. I couldn't stop smiling.

In early September, the 'Just in Case' list made another appearance. After browsing the listed locations, we settled on a November holiday to California with a three-day stopover in New York on the way home, where we planned to meet friends.

Bill had a big birthday while we were away (I'm not allowed to say how big!). We had hoped to mark the occasion with a special holiday, but I had been nervous about booking anything until we had my results.

The holiday was spectacular in every way. We relaxed in the sun every day, and I even wore my bikini, deciding to wear my scar with pride. It was my warrior wound, and I was proud of it. Without it, I wouldn't be alive.

By the time we got to New York, we were feeling chilled and ready to party with our friends, in honour of that extra special birthday. When we raised our glasses to Bill, we also toasted my health. I had come full circle.

I accept that for as long as I live, my life will feel very year to year.

Every year, I will have a trip to Basingstoke, with the uncertainty of scan results.

Maybe I will always feel a slight panic when I get a twinge in my tummy, and maybe not.

I will always be a cancer survivor, but I am coming to terms with my new normal.

Cancer has given me a gift, an appreciation of the now, of the moment.

Every moment I am on this Earth is a gift, a miracle.

I love life.

I love being me.

I will never, ever, lose sight of that again.

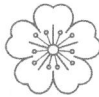

Epilogue: The Beauty of Me

I no longer judge or seek perfection in myself, or others.
It's a waste of energy.
No one is perfect.

I don't need designer labels or fancy possessions to feel special.
It is the quality within me, warts and all, that is important.

I don't need to worry about cancer coming back and killing me.
Dying is a part of living.
When death comes, I will have made the most of every moment.

I don't need to worry about bad stuff happening.
Life will deal its cards.
If I am meant to be here, my instincts will guide me and keep me safe.

I don't focus on what I don't have today,
because I appreciate everything I do have.

I don't need to wait to be happy.
I can be happy today.

The Beauty of Me is just as I am…

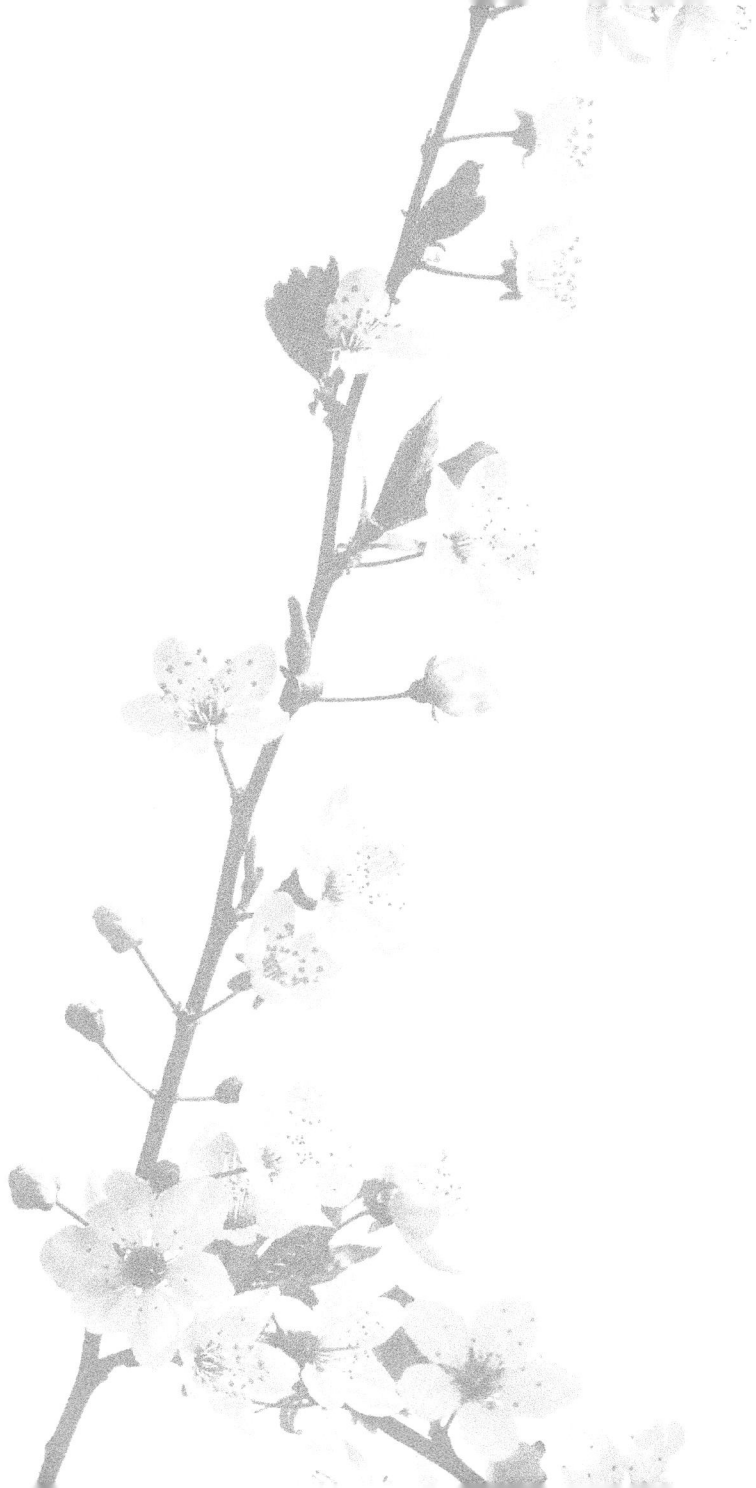

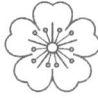

Afterword

I don't quite remember the moment I felt I had become a whole person, as opposed to a fragmented collection of pieces that morphed into a new face for every occasion.

Something shifted, though, which eventually inspired me to share my journey; the long, heart-wrenching path to discover who I really am.

The Beauty of Me was a pipedream at the beginning; something which could be amazing, but was perhaps too aspirational, just out of reach. That is because until I found love and peace within myself, the story couldn't be finished.

I wonder how many people are on the same path, feeling the pressure, putting on a mask, yet go on, year after year, a masquerade of faces and personas?

If you feel trapped inside yourself, I hope this book has encouraged you to take a step back and explore who you really are, settling the demons that can hijack us in any space, at any time.

With a sense of calm fulfilment, I look towards the future with gratitude, optimism and hope. All is exactly as it should be.

In 2026, we are set to do our trip of all trips: the pipedream! A holiday to Australia. We call it Operation Koala Bear.

A promise is a promise after all…

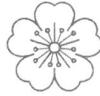

Acknowledgements

I never thought, in a million years, that I would be writing acknowledgements for my own book. That is because I never believed I could write. I have always loved reading, but a book was something other people did!

I have heard people say, "There is a book in everyone."

I believe that now. I had so much I wanted to say, but I also knew I wasn't ready to put pen to paper, and, in my experience, things don't tend to happen in life until they are ready to.

On that note, I want to acknowledge myself for being ready and getting it done. I took on the challenge and put in the time to make this dream become real.

I couldn't have done it without the loving support of my husband, Bill. He has been my anchor through so much, particularly my cancer journey. He believed in me all along. His encouragement and kindness are unwavering and unlimited. Thank you, Darling.

Ross, I can't wait for you to read the book, as I know how much you appreciate books and the freedom of true authenticity. Thank you for giving me plenty of gentle nudges to stick at it during your visits over the last couple of years. You are a wonderful stepson, and I love you dearly.

Jane, we have been through so much as sisters, warts and all. I know that whatever is going on for you, when I need you, you are there. We don't see each other much, but we make it count when we do. Thank you, sis, you are one in a million. I love you.

Maria Iliffe-Wood, IW Press Ltd, thank you. You are a daily inspiration. You took me seriously and saw what was inside me and what needed to come out and be shared with the world. You have mentored me with a gentle kindness and compassion built on a solid foundation of respect and constructive challenge. You have been there every step of the way in my writing journey over the last five years to make this book a reality. Thank you, Maria, with all my heart.

My thank yous would not be complete without a huge shout out to the whole publishing team. Thank you Lisa Mendes, for your efficient and constructive proofreading and to Catherine Williams for your expert formatting. Iain Hill, thank you for creating the gorgeous front cover design. You listened and made my mental vision real. I love it, thank you.

Jacqueline Hollows, my dear friend, life mentor and sister in spirit! You, too, have been an inspiration. A successful and established author in your own right, you have never stopped believing in me. Thank you so much for all your love and support. It means the world.

I want to acknowledge all my close girlfriends, too.

Ann, you have been my best friend since we were seven and have always had my back, whatever life throws our way. We are a team and always will be. Thank you. I love you very much.

To the great girlfriends I have met in more recent village years: Pam, Naomi, Helena and many more (you know who you are). You all ask me regularly how I am getting on with the book, and I love you all for encouraging me to keep going and to believe in myself. I can't wait for you to read it. We will raise a glass of bubbles together to celebrate!

Finally, I want to acknowledge that without the skill and care of my surgeon, Mr Tom Cecil and his support team at the Basingstoke Hampshire Clinic, I wouldn't be here today and *The Beauty of Me*, would never have been written. Your expertise and knowledge of my rare cancer saved my life. A million thank yous. You and your team are amazing, and I will never be able to thank you enough.

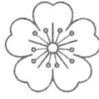

About the Author

I am Lizzie Gardner, a working woman in my mid-fifties.

I work full-time as a leadership consultant and mentor, and live in rural Buckinghamshire with my husband, Bill, and our golden retriever, Lexi.

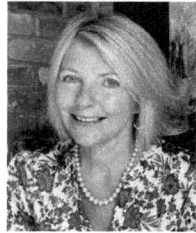

I am step-mum to Ross, sister to Jane, and a devoted auntie to my niece and nephew, Annie and Jacob.

Walking, wildlife and travelling are my passions; each gives me endless opportunity for connection, joy and freedom.

My passion for writing manifested itself during the pandemic when I signed up for an online creative writing course with Maria Iliffe-Wood. Maria helped me believe that anything was possible, and I threw myself into the course, knowing from the very first session that I wanted to write my memoir.

What I didn't know at the beginning was that writing would give me the key to unlock an emotional gateway. It has allowed me to revisit a lifetime of my most treasured, but also most challenging and painful memories.

Like lots of people, I have enjoyed many wonderful things

in my life, but I have also had to navigate some harrowing curveballs in pursuit of finding my true self and a feeling of inner peace.

I am blessed in many ways, and I've also spent years battling anxiety, hijacked by my overthinking and feelings of never being quite good enough.

I guess that's what being human is all about!

It's how we get through it, and what we learn along the way, that shapes us and can even make or break us.

I have had many insights over the years. I treasure each one. They are all special pieces of the jigsaw which together create the big picture – the whole me.

Now is my time to share my search for my truth.

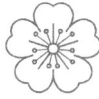

CONNECT WITH LIZZIE

Thank you for reading *The Beauty of Me*. I do hope you enjoyed it.

I would love you to leave a review on your platform of choice.

If you have any questions about anything in the book, please get in touch. I would love to hear from you.

Email: lizziegardner074@gmail.com

For more information about Pseudomyxoma Peritonei, please see Cancer Research UK.